Praise for

'A beautiful invitation to rec[...]
that flows within and between every one of us'
– Kate Raworth, economist and author of *Doughnut
Economics*

'Hrund's book is truly a gift to the world. I am grateful
to her for writing it. It's a practical guide on how
to become your best self and lead with purpose and
authenticity in an increasingly disorderly world'
– Emma Sky OBE, founding director of Yale's
International Leadership Center

'*InnSæi* is the book – and the concept – that today's
world is yearning for' – April Rinne, author of *Flux: 8
Superpowers for Thriving in Constant Change*

'*InnSæi* . . . provides a compass, grounding, and framework
that each human being needs and is capable of without
exception' – HRH Dr Anjhula Mya Singh Bais Chair,
International Board, Amnesty International

'*InnSæi* is both poetic and practical. A treasure trove of
insights, illuminations and exercises that will help you
think, feel and be differently' – Gemma Mortensen,
Co-Creator New Constellations

Praise for InnSæi:

'Profound and practical, deftly observed and beautifully written' – Lindsay Levin, founder of Leaders' Quest and TED Countdown

'The book perfectly captures how we need to rediscover the world around us and deepen our sense of belonging and connection to planet Earth through simple but regular practices. A great read' – Tom Rivett-Carnac OBE, co-author of *The Future We Choose*

'The exercises didn't just teach me to listen to my intuition, but taught me *how* to listen to my intuition again, and when to trust it' – Louis VI, rapper and filmmaker

'*InnSæi* provides deep wisdom and practical guidelines for anyone who seeks to show authentic leadership in our world today' – Paul Polman, co-founder IMAGINE

'This book is full of actionable wisdom: the earlier you read it, the longer it will be a source of warmth and inspiration that will stay with you for a lifetime' – Andrea Bandelli, former executive director of The Science Gallery International

Hrund Gunnsteinsdóttir is an Icelandic sustainability leader, advisor, speaker, writer and filmmaker who brings together ideas and people across sectors and disciplines to inspire creative mindsets and constructive solutions. A firm believer that change starts from within, she draws on her personal and global experience ranging from post-conflict reconstruction and development with the UN, to innovation, investments, filmmaking, nongovernmental and nonprofit organisations, writing and the arts.

She is a trusted advisor to leaders, businesses and universities, financial institutions and nonprofits and is the Co-Director and Script Writer of the documentary film *InnSæi – The Sea Within*, shown worldwide on Netflix, Amazon, vimeo and other streaming services. Hrund sits on the Advisory Council at Yale's International Leadership Center and has been recognised for her leadership by the Icelandic Ocean Cluster, as a Yale World Fellow, a World Economic Forum Young Global Leader and Cultural Leader. She has studied at Stanford, Harvard Kennedy School, LSE, Yale University, Oxford Business School and the University of Iceland.

INNSÆI

ICELANDIC WISDOM
FOR TURBULENT TIMES

HRUND GUNNSTEINSDÓTTIR

Lagom

First published in the UK by Lagom
An imprint of Bonnier Books UK
4th Floor, Victoria House,
Bloomsbury Square,
London, WC1B 4DA

Owned by Bonnier Books
Sveavägen 56, Stockholm, Sweden

Hardback – 9781788708753
Trade Paperback – 9781785124198
Ebook – 9781788708760
Audio – 9781788708777

A CIP catalogue of this book is available from the British Library.

Designed by EnvyDesign Ltd
Printed and bound in Great Britain by Clays Ltd, Elcograf S.p.A

1 3 5 7 9 10 8 6 4 2

Lagom is an imprint of Bonnier Books UK
www.bonnierbooks.co.uk

I dedicate this book to my daughters Rán and Sif
and the younger generations.
And to you, the reader, whoever you are.
— This one's for you.
I hope you enjoy immersing yourself in the world
of InnSæi, it's a great place to be in, I think.
Be brave and keep your heart open.

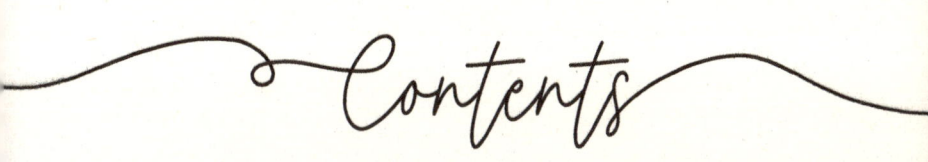

Contents

An Introduction to InnSæi

This book is a love letter, an ode to the magnificent, complex, largely incomprehensible but fascinating world that exists within us all, our InnSæi, meaning *the sea* within us. It explores how we can immerse ourselves beautifully in this inner world, in order to feel regenerated and reconnect with the world around us. It is based on the belief that the more we navigate life with a strong inner compass, aligned to our InnSæi, the more we can become part of the beautiful, generous world that lies outside us. In the words of the planetary scientist and astronomer Carl Sagan: 'The cosmos is also within us. We're made of star stuff. We are a way for the cosmos to know itself.' What we find inside us, in our spirit, is projected on to the world around us.

I love the alchemy of words and the way they can help

us make sense of things. InnSæi, the Icelandic word for intuition, poetically captures the nature of the world within us. It has three meanings: *the sea within*; *to see within*; and *to see from the inside out*. The *sea within* implies dynamic movement; this inner world cannot be put into boxes because then it ceases to flow. To *see within* means to know yourself well enough to be able to put yourself into other people's shoes and make connections that constantly regenerate you. And finally, to *see from the inside out* implies a strong inner compass, which enables you to navigate and create your own path in the ever-changing ocean of life.

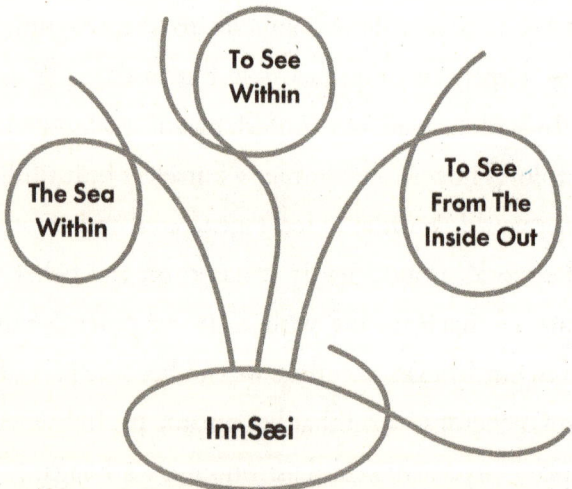

InnSæi is a watery word, which makes this a watery book. This book speaks of oceans, ice-floes, underwater exploration, compasses, the flow of information and the rising of sap in trees. It draws on many of the marvellous functions found in nature's complex ecosystems, and the behaviour of its tiniest beings. The world of InnSæi and intuition is largely intangible and borderless. It may therefore be hard for quantitative, science-based research to measure and quantify; but it is no less important for us to acknowledge, celebrate and befriend. InnSæi follows a different logic from the rational, tangible, conscious, problem-solving approaches that are easily replicated and taught in standard ways. This book unfolds how InnSæi's intelligence is expressed through the whole body: skin, spine, nervous system, brain, heart, gut and senses. As you read on, you will often be reminded of how everything is interconnected, that we are mostly made of the same stuff as stars, that recent scientific findings – in the fields of human genetics, the detection of brainwaves and the electromagnetic fields of our bodies – show that it is not at all clear where you end and I begin. Both human beings and planet Earth have boundaries we cannot cross without threatening our ability to regenerate. InnSæi encompasses all this, and when we deeply connect with InnSæi we embody this understanding of ourselves and our place in the world. It changes the way we act and project on to the world.

I didn't gain real knowledge of InnSæi until I had followed my dreams out into the big wide world, collapsed, lost hope and experienced great pain, before finding a path to healing and self-rediscovery. During my darkest hours, when I was in my late twenties, I could never have imagined that this pain would take me to places where I would meet the most amazing people, that I would create a university program, and that our documentary film based on InnSæi would be shown worldwide. I could not have imagined that RuPaul would tweet about our film *InnSæi – the Sea Within* (subtitled *The Power of Intuition* in North America), that people would tattoo their bodies with InnSæi or design incredible works of art inspired by the sea within.

This book spans centuries, rediscovering the world around us, by celebrating and exploring the world within. It is made up of personal stories from around the globe, including my own, and blends wisdom from different cultures, from science and the arts.

InnSæi can lie dormant if we ignore it or try to silence it; but our very lives depend on being connected to it. When we align with InnSæi, we activate it. My story – about hitting a wall and losing hope – is by no means unique; it is an experience shared with many people from all walks of life. For a while, nothing around me felt solid; and life was incredibly hard, lonely, dark and hopeless. Eventually I found my way back to me, deep within, my truest place of safety. I learnt to connect with and navigate the universe inside me through physical exercises, by delving into science, philosophy, literature, ancient wisdom, writing and simple but constant practices.

Over the past 20 years, InnSæi has given me the courage to follow my inner compass wherever it wants to take me. For this I am extremely grateful. I have had close to thirty different roles in my career so far. I have been a filmmaker, a consultant, a poet, a statistician, a school principal, a playwright, an entrepreneur, an activist, a dreamer, an artistic director, a managing director, a founder, a chair of boards, a what-have-you. But the only role I truly relate to is simply being myself, Hrund, an artist at heart, a visionary and someone who can turn ideas into reality. I would also feel comfortable saying I was a healer, a warrior of light and a sorcerer. It depends how I feel on any given day – there's so much freedom in that. There are many ways to see the world; this book is how I see it.

This book is for those of us who want to explore and be present in the world within, so that we may deepen our sense of belonging, our relationship to ourselves, other people and planet Earth.

Chapter 1 'What is InnSæi?' looks at the different ways we define intuition, according to various schools of thought, cultures and disciplines. We explore the cultural origins of InnSæi, what it really means, what blurs and blocks it, and why it became my holy grail to connect with it and find my bearings again. I share moments from my life and upbringing, and we get a deeper understanding of InnSæi through stories of people from different backgrounds, on their individual journeys. We discover that InnSæi, based on experience and expertise, brings out the highest possible human intelligence. It turns out that a single word can open up the world to us in a whole new way, if we truly embody its meaning in our lives. InnSæi picks up information through every part of our bodies, so this chapter also alerts us to the myriad ways in which we can attend to the world, and prepares us to make use of the tools, tips and exercises offered throughout this book.

In Chapter 2, 'The Healing Power of InnSæi', we'll explore what it means to lose our connection to InnSæi and eventually relocate it. We all go through traumas in our lives. No matter how big or small our trials, they are *our* experiences and they shape us. This chapter shows us how we can emerge from painful experiences as stronger, more compassionate, wiser human beings. I share my own story of how darkness forced me to connect within, as I had nowhere else to go. It took me a while to emerge from that darkness and I wasn't sure if I'd come out merely existing or fully alive.

We can befriend pain through the myth of Inanna, the ancient Mesopotamian goddess of life and death, which teaches us important lessons about how pain can deepen our humanity and help us grow wiser. Using a glacier as a metaphor, our pain either gets frozen within us; or, if we can own it, forgive and let go, our pain melts and evaporates. Reconnecting to InnSæi shifted the way I pay attention and helped me make life-changing decisions. It helped me understand that when we perceive and interpret the world as fragmented, bureaucratic and siloed, this is what it begins to feel like. Instead of staying in that divided world, I wanted to reconnect within, to join people and the world around me, to be present, brave and generous in spirit. This chapter also includes insights from people who know from experience that they are their own healers; the more we connect within and heal our inner world, the more we can relate to and achieve in the world around us.

In Chapter 3, 'The Sea Within', we dive into our borderless and dynamic inner world, which is constantly flowing and helping us make new connections. The ocean is the oldest metaphor for consciousness; and while our knowledge of both is quite limited, they have much in common that helps explain the workings of the sea within and how best to tap into it. Sometimes the best way to activate and align with InnSæi is to immerse ourselves in an activity, which makes us lose track of time and place and reach a state of flow.

The world we live in is complex, fast-changing and non-linear, and – metaphorically speaking – it has a lot in common with the ocean that covers 70 per cent of the Earth's surface. Uncertainty is the only constant, and the unpredictability of tide and waves challenges us to be conscious of where we go and how we get there. The best way to navigate the ocean of life is to become familiar with the sea within. We have to keep our head above the surface in order not to drown; and then we need to decide which direction to go in. Self-awareness and emotional intelligence are important, both to help us relate to others and to access our InnSæi. The word *emotion* means 'to stir, move or agitate'. Let the ocean stir, move and agitate you, but don't let it drown you. Don't *be* the sea – *navigate* it. We need navigation skills, but we need to base our navigation on our inner compass. If not, we risk getting burnt out, losing our way, feeling drained and exhausted, and living the values of others instead of our own.

The last two chapters explain how to harness InnSæi and put it into practice. In Chapter 4, 'To See Within', we put the spotlight on the world inside us, explore its beautiful and sometimes messy landscapes, learn to see through the multiple filters inside us and around us, including the fears, wishes and biases that can block and skew our ability to connect to InnSæi. We continue to deepen our understanding of attention and how it offers us a gateway to InnSæi and a launch pad for a paradigm shift that starts from within. This chapter views our attention as an extremely scarce and precious commodity in a trillion-dollar market. We need to make sure we are aware and in control of how we attend to the world because our impressions inform our InnSæi; otherwise market forces will hijack our attention and distort our perceptions, thoughts and actions. This chapter frames the different ways in which we can chose to attend to the world and offers five rituals that can help us clear the path to InnSæi, take a more mindful ownership of it, activate our creative capacity and open ourselves up to the world around us.

Finally, Chapter 5, 'To See From the Inside Out', brings together much of what we have discussed in the previous chapters, proposing a framework that helps us implement InnSæi in our lives in a practical way. I call this modern navigation tool 'the two rhythms and a strong inner compass'. The human spirit has its own circulation system which it constantly needs to renew and evolve. We also know that InnSæi is embodied and has its own rhythmic ebbs and flows. The better we harness these natural rhythms, the more creative, intelligent and grounded we can become.

In this chapter, we therefore explore how to function in the interplay of the two apparently opposing rhythms – the creative and rational, the intuitive and analytical, the subjective, experienced and sensed versus the calculated, planned and organised. We seek to balance these two rhythms in order to bring out our finest intelligence, well-being, imagination and compassion. The two rhythms and a strong inner compass enable us to stay aligned with and strengthen our dynamic InnSæi, keep our energy and spirit regenerated and our hearts open as we navigate our ocean, through storms and moments of stillness. This chapter dives deeper into how we can make a state of flow a part of our everyday lives. It explores how a sense of awe is worth the world when it comes to shifting our patterns of thinking and becoming more generous, creative and kind.

Our generations are faced with huge challenges that not only defy man-made borders and silos of all sorts, but actually threaten our lives on Earth. Never before have we needed human superpowers like creativity, empathy, tolerance and open-mindedness so much. Never before have we needed the vivid imaginations of so many to create a sustainable future for all. These superpowers are threatened by our modern over-emphasis on rational thinking, algorithms, the way we are constantly bombarded with information, distraction and insecurities, and our increasing levels of burnout, anxiety and stress. Our best hope for a brighter tomorrow lies in shifting our centre of gravity and reconnecting within, to other beings and the natural world.

There are some people who think they belong to the world and other people who think the world belongs to them. But the world was here long before us, and we need to guard against our power outstripping our wisdom and continued existence. We now have access to technology and scientific engineering that was once beyond our wildest dreams, but we need to regain the precious balance between our inner and outer worlds, and the existential connection between us and nature.

We tend to rely on and admire what is external to us. However, the more we rely on externalities, the more we end up living in our heads and not as whole human beings. We must remember that technology and science are a means to an end, and that end should be thriving ecosystems and thriving beings (including human beings). If we lose touch with the natural world, we cease to be inspired; we merely exist and we care less. That is why being tuned in to InnSæi is so important. It lights us up and enables us to create a cosmos out of chaos, by finding our soul's frequency.

InnSæi helps us venture into the void – to see what we can't usually see and to hear what we cannot usually hear – in the spirit of the ancient Polynesian navigators. I have written this book because I believe InnSæi is a much-needed superpower in a world where we place many demands on ourselves, where life can feel incredibly fast, intense and stressful, and – given the state of the planet that is our home – there is no way of knowing how the future will unfold. Both the planet and the human race are now asking for a different, more humane and eco-centric (rather than ego-centric) compass to navigate us into the years to come. The change we want to see in the world starts within us. Systems do not have minds of their own; it is individuals and groups who can make real changes. I believe InnSæi can be a driving force for a thriving world and greater well-being, both personally and collectively.

The art of *InnSæi* encourages you to immerse yourself beautifully in the world within, in order to open up the world around you.

Chapter 1

What is InnSæi?

Intuition is this tremendous library that everyone has inside them. We have the ability to use that library. We are fluent in what it says. Are we going to use that information to make the wisest decisions we can, not only the smartest decisions we can?

DANIEL SHAPIRO, SPEAKING IN THE
DOCUMENTARY FILM INNSÆI

Intuition, or InnSæi, was the key to my journey back to me, and from there, out into the world, where I felt I belonged, connected and aligned. While InnSæi exists within all human beings, you would be surprised to discover how differently we regard it, depending on our languages, disciplines and schools of thought.

The Cambridge Dictionary defines intuition as 'an ability to understand or know something immediately, based on feelings rather than facts'. This sense of knowing that something is either off or feels totally right is familiar to all of us. It's that gut feeling or instinct we have all experienced – Malcolm Gladwell calls it 'the power of thinking without thinking' in his book *Blink* (2005).

Much research has been done and much has been written about intuition in recent years, and various ideas and theories have emerged. Some researchers see intuition as a psychological and spiritual concept, referring to an innate, unconscious wisdom. At the other extreme, intuition is viewed as the key to intellectual genius or its opposite – an irrational impulse that we should not rely on.

After years of personal inquiry, research, practice and conversations all over the world, mostly in English, about intuition, I saw the Icelandic word for intuition, InnSæi, as if I was seeing it for the first time. I was finally able to *embody* its meaning and everything fell into place. InnSæi is a poetic word, rooted in natural forces. It describes a deep, innate sense of intuition, which connects us to ourselves, each other, and the world around us. There are many ways to explain the world – this book explores how we can do it through the lens of InnSæi.

* **Alignment** is when your body, mind and soul are synchronised; and you are tuned in to your InnSæi.

* You feel grounded in yourself; and you navigate with your own inner compass.

* Alignment enables you to function and act with ease and it can be a goal in itself.

* If you are aligned with a particular role, task or journey, it feels as if everything is unfolding as it should.

KEEP A JOURNAL
Keep a journal close at hand. You will need to use it and savour its contents as you read this book and try the various exercises.

The threefold meaning of InnSæi

Modern Icelandic comes from old Norse, the language spoken by the Vikings. While Icelandic has changed and evolved over time, like other languages, modern speakers can still read the oldest preserved texts written in the 12th and 13th centuries. In Icelandic, we don't adopt foreign words (like *computer* or *smartphone*) and use Icelandic phonetics to make up equivalents, as some other languages do. Instead, we create new words for new ideas or technological innovations and the words typically describe the function of that particular thing or idea. For example, the Icelandic word for a computer is *tölva*. It was coined in 1965 by the Icelandic scholar, writer and ambassador, Sigurdur Nordal, from *tala* (meaning 'number') and *völva* (meaning 'prophetess'). *Völva* in Old Norse and Icelandic is a female shaman or seer – a woman who sees into the future –and the female seer is a recurring motif in Norse mythology. 'Icelandic is therefore a relatively transparent language, unlike many other languages,' says Gudrun Nordal, Director of the Institute of Árni Magnusson for Icelandic Studies and granddaughter of the late Sigurdur Nordal.

Although the first use of the word intuition in English texts is from around the 15th century, InnSæi didn't find its way into the written Icelandic language until the early 20th century, for example when a book by the theosophist Annie Besant was translated from English by Sig. Kristófer Pétursson, published in 1916 and titled *Lífsstiginn*.

The key to unlocking the meaning of the word InnSæi lies in how the word is put together, which is why I prefer to write InnSæi (pronounced 'in-sy-ay') with a capital S and I. However, if you look up the word in an Icelandic dictionary, you will find it written all in lower case: innsæi.

As mentioned in the Introduction, InnSæi has a threefold, poetic meaning. It merges two words: *Inn* (translated as 'inside' or 'into') and *Sæi* (derived from the verb 'to see' but also evoking *sær*, the word for 'sea'). In short, InnSæi is your inner guide, the voice of your soul; and in spheres where you have expertise, it can bring out your highest intellectual capacity.

The sea within conjures up the borderless nature of our inner world. It is constantly moving and making new connections. It goes beyond words. It is a world of vision, feelings and imagination. It is home to the undercurrents of emerging directions in life, a sense of alignment and instincts about important decisions even before we can express them in words. The sea within cannot be put into boxes or silos, because then it ceases to flow.

To see within is to see inside yourself – to know yourself well enough to witness your own creativity, core beliefs and humanity, including your imperfections, strengths, biases, fears and vulnerabilities. When you see within yourself, you are more able to empathise, speak your truth and live authentically.

And finally, *to see from the inside out* means being aligned with your inner compass. You are mindfully present in the world, and your heart, spine, head and gut are aligned. In a world that is full of uncertainty, opportunities, speed and ceaseless attempts to numb our senses and hijack our attention, a strong inner compass gives you clarity, focus and resilience. It enables you to better navigate your individual path across the ocean of life.

My InnSæi roots

I grew up in Iceland and although we didn't use the word InnSæi that much, it was always there somehow, lingering in the air and stimulating my imagination. As a child, I spent a lot of time in nature, exploring the lava fields close to my home or running away from the trolls that I imagined were out to get me and take me away from my family. I would roam for hours there and lose all track of time.

As a family of six, we travelled around Iceland in the summer months, camping or going on day trips whenever we had the chance and the weather permitted. I remember walking home by myself from a very young age, around six years old. On winter's nights, after a long day with friends, I was never afraid of the dark. When I lay outside in the snow and looked up at the starry night sky, I felt most at home in the big world out there. I had imaginary conversations with the stars and felt we were sharing a moment.

My mother is an artist, and has been a self-taught pianist from an early age, who went on to get an arts degree in her forties and founded an art gallery with four other female artists. She would fill the house with beautiful music, playing the white piano in the living room, in between her busy work schedule. Meanwhile, my siblings and I would be drawing, painting, sewing or making things around the house, sometimes staying up way past our bedtimes.

Before I even knew how to spell, I would pretend to write short stories on my grandmother's typewriter. When I was eight years old, I announced that I was planning to publish my first book. I knew how I wanted it to look – a brown leather-bound hardback volume – but I was less clear about the storyline. Sometimes my siblings would make fun of me, which hurt me deeply; so much so that I would sometimes lock myself in my bedroom for what felt like hours and refuse to speak to anyone except my mum who guarded my imagination by listening to my ideas and taking them seriously.

At the age of nine I founded a company with my childhood friend Edda. We called it 'le Crabe' because we had found a stack of red stickers with a picture of a white crab and the letters *le Crabe* written below it. My dad gave us an out-of-date cheque book which added considerable gravitas to our business, at least in appearance. In reality, all we did was exchange letters with more than a hundred pen pals from around the world. On the days when we didn't receive letters, we assumed there had been a mistake and marched to the post office together to ask if they could double-check whether any letters had arrived for us.

Around the age of ten, I asked Dad if I could have an office space at his tyre company, something that felt like the next logical step on my journey. He politely refused my request and did his best not to laugh at me. Dad built two of our homes and a company with my granddad, which he ran for decades. He was a handball player who became captain of the national handball team in the 1970s; and he was later selected for the national golf team for senior players. In short, I was raised by parents whose combined skills and passions embraced sports, arts, business and entrepreneurship – all areas that require imagination and creativity and thousands of hours of training and practice. I have three siblings and at home there was a lot of talk about the importance of hard work and we all had a rock-solid faith instilled in us that we could do anything we wanted if we set our minds to it.

The word InnSæi is a universe on its own

Words matter. Just as every individual is a universe on their own, so is each word. I love the way words help us capture meaning. We use words to process and frame what we perceive, experience and imagine. They emerge through clues that we see when we pay attention. We create words to describe the world as we experience it – and there's so much we need to express.

Putting words to what we sense and feel may take days, weeks or years and yet a new word is created every

98 minutes, amounting to 5,400 new words per year, according to the Global Language Monitor. InnSæi is a poetic word that offers insights into the ebb and flow of the sea within us, how we connect to it, to each other and the natural world. It acknowledges that complexity and simplicity co-exist, and everything is interconnected, and helps us see the world that way.

For centuries, the complex interconnectedness of living systems has been explained through science, philosophy and spiritualism. This interconnectedness often goes beyond what we can measure or see with the naked eye. For instance, we cannot take apart complex natural systems – like the Amazon rainforest, relationships, the human body or mind – and then put them back together and expect them to work as they did before. In contrast, we *can* dismantle and reassemble a complicated mechanical structure, like a car or a machine. When we navigate with our InnSæi, we gain a fuller understanding of the huge difference between machines and nature.

InnSæi combines ancient wisdom and modern science

Whether we dive into ancient spiritual or philosophical traditions or modern quantum physics, we gain a deeper understanding of how everything is interconnected and that when things or particles interconnect and affect something else, they begin 'to exist', be real and alive. This is very different from the more abstract, siloed approach to reality we are accustomed to encountering in education and at work. The way we connect the myriad of dots is very much up to our InnSæi. Let's explore a few examples.

At a young age, I was introduced to Paganism at school, which taught me that humans are an integral part of the ecosystem; that humans are a part of nature, along with other animals, trees, stones, plants and everything else that is of this Earth. In other words, the way we interact with the ecosystem helps create and shape our lives.

Paganism became even more magical when one of our teachers told us that when we are alone in nature and speak our wishes or thoughts out loud, a stone will hear us. And the stone will tell a bird and the bird will tell a tree. With all its branches and thousands of leaves, we can only imagine how many birds the tree will tell it to, creating ripple effects beyond our wildest dreams. In this way, the natural world transforms our thoughts and wishes into reality.

However, this also worried me a bit because it meant I needed to be careful about the thoughts I had, and my fears, hopes and wishes, as they would all come true. As the old saying goes, 'Be careful what you wish for, be mindful of your thoughts.' The ancient Pagan religion first taught me that my thoughts and beliefs shaped words, and words expressed my experiences. When crafted together, words make stories, stories create narratives, and narratives shape human history.

CATCH YOUR THOUGHTS

According to a study carried out at Queen's University Canada, humans have around 6.5 thoughts per minute, or about 6,000 per day, assuming that we sleep for 8 hours (and discounting any thoughts we have while sleeping).

- We often have a lot of 'noisy' thoughts buzzing around in our minds, which we mostly don't pay attention to. But if you start noticing your thoughts and writing them down, it's a good first step towards clarity of thought, which helps you access InnSæi.
- Try jotting your thoughts down in your journal. Don't think about it – just write them down. They don't have to be described in detail.

These ideas are echoed in the influential work of 21st-century historian Yuval Noah Harari. In his groundbreaking book *Sapiens: A Brief History of Humankind* (2015), he argues that story-telling shapes civilisations. According to Harari, story-telling not only enables us to imagine and rationalise things, but to do so *collectively*. On an individual level, our thoughts and beliefs define who we become. When we *collectively* believe in a narrative, that story shapes our world. In today's world, where powerful market forces are specifically designed to hijack our attention, we need to be more determined than ever to stay in control of our own minds and the narrative we live by.

We can also find traces of Paganism in quantum physics, which is one of our most successful ways of explaining the world around us. Quantum theory has clarified the structure of the periodic table, the functioning of the sun, the colour of the sky, the formation of galaxies and much more. Based on this theory, we have been able to develop technologies ranging from computers to lasers.

The fascinating thing about quantum theory is that it explains reality not by means of single particles or units, but by the relationships between them and how they affect each other. Nevertheless, a lot of physical systems remain unexplained by quantum theory, and this presents a huge challenge for a lot of scientists who believe that what we cannot measure does not exist. According to Carlo Rovelli, professor of physics and the author of *Helgoland: Making Sense of the Quantum Revolution* (2021), reality is what happens when particles touch and interconnect. Writing in *The Guardian*, Rovelli says: 'Perhaps it really does reveal to us the deep structure of reality, where a property is no more than something that affects something else. Properties are the effects of interactions. A good scientific theory, then, should not be about how things "are", or what they "do": it should be about how they affect one another.'

This way of explaining and seeing the world is echoed in both Eastern and Western traditions, writes Rovelli in *The Guardian*. The ancient Greek philosopher Plato and the Buddhist philosopher Nagarjuna wrote over 2000 years ago that the definition of being is simply action. In other words, if something can affect something else, it means that it exists.

Those who consciously align with InnSæi understand that knowledge, experience, stimuli and emotions touch, interconnect and accumulate in patterns inside us in a myriad of ways. Through this multifaceted interaction with the world around us, a 'knowing' emerges. We cannot explain exactly how this happens, but with practice and experience we learn to accept the unexplained part of the process, as we harness and trust our InnSæi more and more. InnSæi becomes our inner compass and enables us to embody the ecosystem thinking that we so desperately need to build a flourishing future for ourselves and the planet. When we innately navigate with InnSæi at the core, it changes the way we connect with ourselves, other living beings and the Earth. This means we move from an over-emphasis on siloed, inanimate, abstract and quantifiable thinking to a more animate, holistic and sensory interaction with reality. Finding a balance between the abstract and rational, and the inner world of InnSæi, we are able to navigate more steadily, wisely and innovatively in our dynamic and constantly evolving world. This enhances our ability to think logically and use our imagination for human and planetary progress.

We all have InnSæi; it's part of being human and alive, whatever our age and gender, and wherever we come from. InnSæi is always there, inside us, and it sharpens our inner compass if we chose to follow it. Turning it on, tuning into it and regularly updating it is up to us.

The trick is to train our attention to witness it evolve before an idea, skill, 'knowing', vision, decision, direction or feeling emerges. On a personal level, we use our InnSæi to make choices, communicate with other people and fall in love. We take a risk when we decide to trust someone or take a leap of faith based on InnSæi that will turn the tide in our lives. On a professional level, we may develop certain skills or even excel in a particular domain, and then we weave InnSæi together with reason and analysis. We begin to learn when to let things sink in and brew and when to be deliberate and execute. InnSæi taps into the 95–99 per cent of our consciousness which lies outside our focused attention. Our focused attention can only take in about 1–5 per cent of all the data we are exposed to. Once we become aware that we attend to the world not just with our heads, but with our whole being and all our senses, we can start to embody InnSæi. To explain this, I'll share stories of my mother, a BMX rider, a former Iraqi fighter pilot and a French horse trainer and the different ways they each use their InnSæi.

Music and flow

My mother was a self-taught pianist and she could play any popular song or classical piece of music we asked her to, as long as she had heard it herself. She just sat down and played – and became one with the piano. It didn't happen overnight; it took lots of practice and dedication. This is how skilled intuition, or InnSæi, works says Gerd Gigerenzer, psychologist, author and former Director of the Max Planck Institute: "You practise deliberately and then it goes into a different domain, the unconscious," he explains. You practise each note for hours and hours, but the music only begins when you are no longer conscious of how your fingers are moving across the keys. In other words, you are immersed in the act of playing – you have become one with the music.

Imagine my mum is playing the piano, totally in the zone, immersed in the music. Then imagine that someone goes up to her and says, 'You are an amazing pianist, how do you play so well?' This instantly makes her lose her rhythm. She starts to consciously think about how she does it and the flow gets disrupted. When we learn a method or a craft we consciously practise it. The skill then gets imprinted in our unconsciousness, the sea within, and we stop consciously thinking how we do it. This shows that tapping into our InnSæi often means switching off our logical brains and letting what we know flow.

Making space for intuition

You get your intuition back when you make space for it, when you stop the chattering of the rational mind.

ANNE LAMOTT, *BIRD BY BIRD: SOME INSTRUCTIONS ON WRITING AND LIFE* (1995)

The human body is intelligent, down to a single cell: it knows, remembers, learns, rehabilitates and adjusts to different scenarios. When Mat Hoffman, an American BMX rider, one of the best vert ramp riders in the history of the sport, suffered from amnesia after a serious fall, it was his body's memory that came to the rescue. Mat's story is discussed during an episode of *Armchair Expert* between the host Dax Shepard and Kelly Slater. Kelly speaks of how

Mat found himself standing at the top of a 14-foot vert ramp at an exhibition he'd been booked for; and when he looked down he felt terrified and didn't know what to do. He literally couldn't remember how to ride his bike. But he decided to take a leap of faith and simply trust his body. In that moment, his mind came back, and his body remembered. We have all had to physically go back to places to remember where we left things or how things were in the past. Likewise, when we cycle or ski after a long gap, we instantly see how our bodies remember and the skill returns.

Intuitive judgement

In 2016 I took a taxi from New Haven to Hartford in Connecticut to do an interview on the *Where We Live* show on WNPR radio. The driver was Mohamad, a former fighter pilot from Iraq, a friendly guy I had got to know through a mutual friend during my time in the US that year. The interview was about our film *InnSæi – the Power of Intuition* which had premiered in the US a few weeks earlier. The drive was about two hours long and, as I prepared for the interview, I asked Mohamad about his experience of intuition when he was a fighter pilot in Iraq.

Mohamad spoke passionately about intuition and gave a very good example of how he had once used it in his professional life. He described being present at a meeting with Iraq's highest-ranking army officials, when they were discussing a critical situation. At one point they turned to him and asked for his opinion on a big decision they had to make. All eyes were on him – it was a stressful moment and he needed to think fast.

Mohamad told me the two things that mattered most in that situation: the first was that he had a lot of experience to base his decision on; and the second was that he had confidence in his intuition in this area. He also knew that his intuition worked best when he had space and quiet in which to think – and that gave him the confidence to ask the officials to please leave the room while he considered their question.

Mohamad's story supports what scientific research has shown. In a situation where there is certainty and 'known knowns', statistics and analysis apply. In situations of uncertainty, it is our InnSæi that works best, especially when it is based on experience and knowledge. In fact, research shows that the latter combination is when we can reach the highest intelligence possible, according to experts like Gerd Gigerenzer. While we wouldn't send a man to the moon based on intuition alone, the more knowledge and experience we have in a certain domain, the more we can rely on our intuitive judgement to enable us to make good decisions.

Trusting our intuition

In *The Matter with Things*, Iain McGilchrist tells a fascinating story about Franck Mourier, the French horse trainer who had all his life been deeply passionate about horses and at university established a complex mathematical model for selecting the best thoroughbreds. He saw himself as very methodical and analytical, and was highly experienced in buying, selling and training racehorses. When he retired he started making a living by going to the races every day and acting as a tipster. He would watch the runners for a few minutes before a race and estimate each horse's chances of winning. One year he had done 1,200 estimates on pieces of paper, kept records and analysis of all the data and discovered that his percentage had been consistently better and more accurate than the market consensus. Through Iain McGilchrist's communication with Franck Mourier and his wife, a few things emerged as lessons about his intuition that are worth highlighting here.

When Franck Mourier let his doubts, distrust, fear of losing and self-blame get in the way of his judgements he would do worse. His challenge was to simply trust what he saw, to trust his intuition. Part of his explanation was that he had always considered himself a scientist who based all his decisions on reason and analysis, and his ability to predict almost without thinking made him suspicious that this was possible – it went against his academic training.

The more Franck Mourier trained being mindful about his intuition and trusting in it, the more he relaxed into his talent, and his wife remarked that he started being more open, talking about his emotions, became more sensitive to the things around him, and more creative too. This changed his role in the family and his relationship with his wife in a whole range of ways for the better. They also noticed he had more need for a long sleep and what also helped were short naps in the car, right before the races started. What is also worth mentioning is that he needed to disassociate himself from 'anything material or financial' during the mornings before the race. 'The best results are achieved when I see it as just a game with no pressure – as if I am going to the races just to enjoy the horses and write the per centages I feel.'

Things that can obstruct InnSæi

* Self-doubts, lack of confidence, fear of losing, self-blame

* Stress

* Material or financial pressure

* Not taking our intuition seriously enough

because it often speaks to us in a gentle and effortless way

* Allowing our biases (mental habits) to dominate our thinking, e.g. preferring what is familiar to what is different

    * Gender biases are common, according to studies by Gerd Gigerenzer and his collaborators (see Notes). For instance, men tend to be less likely to admit publicly that they follow their intuition because it is commonly thought that women are more intuitive and men more rational. Cultural norms have taught us to trust rationality and not intuition, and men over women. But studies show that no matter their gender, everyone has intuition.

    * Another common bias is to choose to act quickly rather than take our time.

    * We are often unaware that some of our perceptions are not objective truths. We need to remember that they are actually our subjective perceptions and they can change, once we have more or different information.

    * A safety bias is the tendency to protect ourselves against loss more than seeking to gain.

* ★ Other biases include stereotyping, over-
  confidence, and anchoring (when we rely
  heavily on one piece of information and neglect
  others, in making final decisions). Confirmation
  bias is when we interpret new information to
  support our pre-existing view and disregard
  other knowledge. The list goes on ...

InnSæi is key to creativity, and creativity is key to innovation, which is what makes economies thrive and organisations competitive. When NASA wanted to make sure they were hiring the most creative minds, they asked Dr George Land and Dr Beth Jarman to develop a test to identify the capacity for creativity and divergent thinking. The test results were shocking. They showed that *98 per cent of five-year-olds fell into the 'genius category of imagination', but this per centage dropped dramatically to 12 per cent for 15-year-olds and only 2 per cent for adults.*

As we go through the school system and join the workforce, our ability to stay aligned with our InnSæi, and to be creative, decreases. This is because the more rational, tangible, conscious problem-solving skills can be taught in standard ways, which is what we do in schools all over the world. These processes are easily replicated, measured, compared and assessed, and this approach seeps into our systems and work processes, where we rely on quantifiable metrics. Meanwhile, the intuitive approach is unconscious, relying on stored memories and loose neural connections over time, thus requiring a more random and patient process for acquisition, writes Wilma Koutstaal in her book *The Agile Mind* (2013). Koutstaal's work supports what has repeatedly been shown, that when we combine unconscious, intuitive ways with analytical, rational conscious methods, we use our highest intelligence and can outperform those who use only the latter.

Seeing, hearing, feeling more

Ours is a culture based on excess, on over-production; the result is a steady loss of sharpness in our sensory experience. What is important now is to recover our senses. We must learn to See more, to Hear more, to Feel more.

SUSAN SONTAG (1933–2004), PHILOSOPHER, WRITER AND POLITICAL ACTIVIST, IN AGAINST INTERPRETATION AND OTHER ESSAYS (1966)

There are many ways in which we can attend to the world and this book focuses on ethical InnSæi that promotes humane and generous ways of being and co-creating. The 2008 recession, which Icelanders called 'the bank collapse', opened the way to new ideas. People were eager to rethink our decision-making systems and open the floodgates of creative and critical thinking for ethical and constructive purposes in a world that seemed to have gone mad.

At that time, I designed and co-created a university diploma module in Iceland, based on what I called 'two rhythms and a strong inner compass', which is the theme of the last chapter in this book. The module essentially trained students in how to effectively combine the rhythms of divergent and convergent thinking, analysis and creativity, reason and InnSæi, in order to sharpen their inner compass.

Given the overflow of information and noisy distraction in today's culture, Susan Sontag's words (written in 1966) now ring truer than ever. Sontag encouraged us to use our sensory intelligence, to put ourselves back into the world, to sense it with our whole being, and to view the spinning of public narratives in news cycles with a critical eye.

She encouraged us to see more, hear more and feel more because she wanted us to access our inner artist, to reawaken our senses to better understand the meaning of things, including the pain of others. Our creativity, authentic leadership and voice in the world all depend on how we use our senses and pay attention. Susan Sontag inspired us to look beyond interpretation and headlines, to get to the core of what it means to be human.

SEE MORE, HEAR MORE, FEEL MORE
- Use your journal to capture what you see, hear and feel.
- Don't judge what your attention picks up, just jot it down.
- As you document each sensation, you are witnessing yourself at that moment.

Susan Sontag has been a big inspiration for my work on InnSæi. In this context, 'to see more' means tuning into our senses and attending to how our whole body picks up clues and data. It is through our bodies that we connect with InnSæi. When our connection to InnSæi is blocked, our direction in life becomes unclear; we swing from one decision or opinion to another; and we start to distrust ourselves.

As Dr Nicole LePera explains in her book *How to Do the Work* (2021), we start to believe the swirling, inhibiting, anxious thoughts in our heads and forget that we can instigate our own thoughts. Our thoughts are not necessarily who we are, writes LePera; we can change how we think. When we believe the unhealthy thoughts in our heads, they weaken us; our mind becomes our worst enemy because it blocks our connection to our inner wisdom and makes it impossible for us to gain clarity and trust our own judgement. It is only when we become more self-aware that we can start to free ourselves from the thoughts that are holding us back.

InnSæi is an embodied feeling, which means that it is transmitted through our whole bodies. Let's explore how our bodies speak to us and help us stay aligned with our InnSæi.

The skin

We'll start with the skin, the outer covering that protects our skeleton, organs, veins, tendons and neurosystem. As the body's biggest organ, the skin plays a vital role in regulating our body temperature, and protecting our muscles, bones and internal organs from infection and disease. Our skin accounts for about 15 per cent of our body weight. We have about 300 million skin cells and we shed 30,000–40,000 dead skin cells every minute of every day. The skin renews itself every 28 days. Our bodies react to a universal electrical field found in other people, objects, in nature and even in the ground we stand on; the hairs on our skin stand up straight in the presence of these electrical fields.

Changes in our skin can sometimes signal changes in our overall health: our skin may look more radiant when we are happy and healthy; and it often looks grey or dry when we are not well. In effect, our skin 'speaks to us' and helps us witness our interaction with our environment. For instance, we may get goosebumps when we feel deeply moved by a piece of music or a loving act. If someone gives you 'chills down your spine' there's a reason for your reaction – and sometimes you may simply be picking up the energy of people in the same room.

PAY ATTENTION TO YOUR SKIN

- Notice what your skin is telling you and jot it down in your journal. This will help you get to know yourself better through your skin.
- You will see patterns emerging and these patterns will help you see what is on the periphery of your focused mind, what your InnSæi is trying to tell you about how you sense people and surroundings.
- Your reactions may differ, depending on the day and the circumstances. Record your state of energy at these moments, if you wish. Things like sleep, food, emotional well-being, whether you feel relaxed, stressed, loved or lonely, can all affect what you pick up with your skin.

*Intuition is not just some pink and fluffy feeling.
Intuition is the awareness of the subtle stuff which
lies outside the focus of attention; the stuff that
we're aware of subliminally, unconsciously.
And if we spend too much time in the stance of
our very focused conscious mind, we will not see
why that should be important; it doesn't seem
to be present, it doesn't seem to matter and one
therefore cuts it out.*

IAIN MCGILCHRIST, PSYCHIATRIST AND AUTHOR, SPEAKING IN
INNSÆI DOCUMENTARY

The senses

Our senses take in millions of items of data every hour of every day. We cannot possibly be aware of all this information without losing our minds. So, while we want to open our senses in order to see more, hear more and feel more, there will also be times when we want to protect our senses from the outside world, to ensure that our access to InnSæi remains intact. In other words, we sometimes consciously and mindfully open our senses, and we sometimes deliberately shut them down, in order to keep our energy balanced and not become overwhelmed.

Attention is vital when tuning into our InnSæi, creativity and mindfulness. We pay attention to a lot of things every single day, but we are very unconscious of *what* we are paying attention to. By 'noticing more what we notice', we start to find out what informs our intuitions. Writing down the things we notice enables us to harness our intuition even more. When we do this, we are allowing the world to come to us; we are turning the light on, so to speak. We start to notice things we didn't notice before, because we weren't truly present. When we start to notice what we notice, we shift our attention to the unconscious, the subtle details of information that linger in the air, waiting for us to discover them. We will explore this further in Chapter 4, but for now it is enough to highlight how 'paying attention to attention' helps us connect to all our senses.

PAY ATTENTION TO WHAT YOU PAY ATTENTION TO, AND WRITE IT IN YOUR JOURNAL

- Jot down in your journal what you notice about or with your senses, using your eyes, ears, body, fingers, feet, skin.
- Notice when you notice the body language of people or animals.
- Don't judge what you notice, just jot it down.
- Simply observe what your senses are picking up. Allow the world to come to you.

When we feel overwhelmed, exhausted, worried or sad, we may feel the need to protect our senses from the outside world in order to restore our energy. Think of it as filling our tank or recharging our body's battery. It's a way of setting our own boundaries and giving ourselves permission to rest, restore our energy and take the time to simply be. This is part of being self-aware as well as expressing self-care and self-love. When we feel lacking in love for ourselves, we should do the work and develop it – because without it, we cannot show love and support to others.

There are many reasons why our nervous system sometimes gets weakened or over-stimulated. We may have gone without enough sleep for some time; we may be suffering from a disease that puts a strain on our system; perhaps there is too much noise at work or at home; or we have simply been under too much stress for other reasons. We may get short of breath or we may want to avoid being in crowded places, which we might otherwise quite enjoy. Environmental over-stimulation means that our senses have taken in more information than our brains can process.

When our nervous system is weak or over-stimulated, it reacts more strongly than normal to stressors. Small stressors or stimuli can therefore evoke relatively big responses. Sounds can feel extra loud, lights brighter, and may we feel that people are demanding too much of our attention and energy. We don't feel as much in control of our focus or energy as we do on a good day. Other symptoms can include loss of sight or double vision, memory loss, loss of feeling or tingling in the body and headaches.

SIMPLE WAYS TO PROTECT A VULNERABLE AND OVER-STIMULATED NERVOUS SYSTEM

The following simple practices can help you restore your nerves and minimise stimulation:

- Wear a cap, a hat or a hoodie to minimise stimulation to the ears, eyes and head.
- Wear noise-cancelling headphones or listen to calming sounds on your headphones if you are going out and about.
- Wear green-tinted glasses; the colour green helps calm your nervous system.
- Go outside and spend time near green grass, leaves, plants and trees, and simply observe their sounds, colours, shapes, patterns and smell.
- Walk barefoot on the ground.
- If you are in a challenging situation at work or in your personal life, and you feel it is soaking up all your energy, imagine seeing it from a distance, from the top of a mountain or looking

down from the sky. If you observe the situation from afar, you don't *become* the situation.

- Meditate – breathe deeply, in and out, focus only on your breath.

'CENTRE YOURSELF'

This is a great meditation for when you feel you are losing yourself in a situation. If you only have five minutes, use them. More is even better. Do it a few times over the course of the day if you feel that is what would be good for you. Show yourself kindness.

- Centering yourself means bringing your mind back into your body. You mindfully let go of thoughts that are taking you away from yourself, so to speak. These are thoughts or worries you may be having about the future or the past, or something that feels too much at the moment.
- Find a comfortable position. Take a few deep breaths and follow your breaths with your mind. Thank your breaths for breathing you.
- While focusing on the breaths, acknowledge your senses, one at a time, with each breath. Your eyes, ears, nose, tongue, whole body and mind.
- Visualise the whole of you and imagine you are sitting peacefully inside a lotus flower or a

beautiful transparent capsule which no one but you can see or enter. This lotus flower or capsule protects your whole being, your senses, from the outside world and stimulation that may feel too much at times.

- As you are breathing inside your protection shield, with your eyes closed, you don't look anymore, you don't listen anymore, you don't think anymore; you just follow your breath and you are comfortable inside your body, your temple, your home.

- Every time you feel lost and that you are no longer yourself, you have been blown away by events. Then it's time to go home to your true self, align your mind with your body and connect with the sea within until it is calm; until you feel anchored inside yourself. Tell yourself: I am safe.

- Your deepest sense of security comes from deep within yourself. When you feel safe, or safer in this mediation, you may like to start by opening your eyes, ears and whole body to the environment around you. As you continue the day, the week, or month, you can imagine being enfolded inside the lotus flower or beautiful capsule as your protection shield which no one else but you can see or enter.

The brain

*The brain is a far more open system than we ever
imagined, and nature has gone very far to help us
perceive and take in the world around us. It has
given us a brain that survives in a changing world
by changing itself.*

NORMAN DOIDGE, PSYCHIATRIST AND AUTHOR, *THE BRAIN
THAT CHANGES ITSELF* (2007)

The brain is the Grand Central Station for processing the
information that our cells, senses, skin and nerves pick up
and interpret every day. Despite the massive amount of
research that's been done on the brain, our knowledge
of its workings is still limited. The average adult brain
weighs about 1.4 kilograms and contains around
75 per cent water. The brain is a vast web of connections,
consisting of 86 to 100 billion neurons, as many as
the stars in our galaxy, embedded in a scaffolding of a
100 billion glial cells and connected by trillions of synapses
or junctions between nerve cells.

If you could hold it in your hand, you would see that
the human brain is a jelly-like mass, easily deformed by
touch, dead and useless when disconnected from the rest
of the body. It's seen as the host of logic and intellect; it

enables us to think, perceive and make sense of things. It receives an immense amount of information via our senses and the neuropathways that run from the gut, heart and vagus nerve to the brain.

Amazingly, the brain is always changing, it adapts to life experiences and enables us to learn new things throughout our lives. It is divided into left and right hemispheres, which have different characteristics when it comes to how we see the world. There are several mini-stations inside this central hub that serve different roles. Some parts of the brain serve us best in times of danger, others when we want to be creative or excel in communicating. We will be exploring this in greater depth later.

We cannot physically see our brains connecting and synchronising but studies show that the heartbeats and brainwaves of couples synchronise when they are close together; and this can also apply to colleagues and friends, and even strangers. Many of us have seen one of our loved ones in a stressful situation, and felt it affect the beating of our own hearts.

The more I read about how we communicate with our bodies, brains and electromagnetic fields, the more I wonder if it is at all clear where I end and you begin. I interviewed Dr Rebekah Granger-Ellis, an expert in neurowellbeing and neurobiology of learning, who confirmed that the boundaries between individual human beings aren't at all clear:

We co-regulate as a species, we are so completely interconnected that our brains are always silently rewiring other brains. We are so socially wired as human beings, attentional, emotional and behavioural, that we register each other's internal states and mirror them. Even just being next to another human being for a short amount of time, our brainwaves and neural populations will begin to synchronise, breathing patterns will mimic one another's, and our heart rates will regulate together. Even our interaction between body and our environment, our Earth and sun, everything we interact with, contains energy, and it moves back and forth between objects all the time. [...] Through a quantum physics lens, we are fractals made of the same particles, our DNA is made up of carbon, hydrogen, oxygen, nitrogen, phosphorus and other trace elements. We share particles and electricity with the sun, and the ground we are standing on regulates our nervous system and cells in complex ways as well.

The heart

*The heart has its reasons, which reason knows
nothing of*

BLAISE PASCAL, FRENCH PHILOSOPHER AND
MATHEMATICIAN (1623–1662)

We have probably all heard the saying 'follow your heart' when we are encouraged to follow our inner voice or sense of purpose. The heart, like the gut, contains an intrinsic nervous system that has both short and long-term memory functions. It is sometimes called our 'second brain' and contains around 40,000 neurons, according to an oft cited study by Dr Armour from 1991. The heart beats before the brain is formed, and continues to beat as long as it has oxygen, even after the brain is dead. The heart pumps blood to the entire circulatory system so that our organs, tissues and cells receive nutrients and oxygen. It also eliminates waste, such as carbon dioxide.

The word courage comes from the Latin root *cor*, meaning 'heart'. When we 'speak from the heart' we speak our truth, we move others and build trust. This isn't just an expression because research shows that, like our brain, the heart secretes oxytocin, the so-called love hormone. According to Thomas R. Verny in *The Embodied Mind*

(2021), oxytocin motivates us to like and empathise with others, and extend and reciprocate trust and cooperation. Feelings of anger and sadness can cause heart failure so we can literally 'die of a broken heart', writes Iain McGilchrist in *The Matter with Things,* citing various studies.

The heart's magnetic field, which is the strongest rhythmic electromagnetic field produced by the human body, not only envelops every cell of the body, but also extends out in all directions into the space around us. The heart's electrical field is about 60 times bigger than the electrical field generated by the brain; and the heart's magnetic field can be measured several metres away from the body by sensitive magnetometers. The expression to 'touch someone's heart' means to instil or awaken something in them. Imagine the ripple effects of a loving heart…

We can all communicate without words, through our body's magnetic fields.

CONNECT WITH YOUR HEART
- Close your eyes and take a few deep breaths; exhale for twice as long as you inhale, if you can.
- Focus on your chest as it moves with each breath.
- Imagine you have a flash light inside your body. Turn it on and start in your head. Use the flash

light to light up your brain inside your skull, the inside of your face, neck and throat; then move down to where you can see your heart beating, strong and healthy, inside your chest.

- Observe it for a moment and honour your heart for what it is and what it does; see how it pumps blood in all directions, to different parts of your body.
- Now place your hand on your chest, and feel the warmth from your healing hand.
- Imagine your heart transforming into a rosebud, or any flower you wish. Observe the rosebud or flower that symbolises your heart. Watch as it opens up to you and the world around you.
- Enjoy this vision and notice if it brings a smile to your face.

The gut

Trust your gut, it knows what your head hasn't figured out yet.
ANONYMOUS

Our gut is home to most of our happiness hormones; it is closely connected to our emotional and physical well-being and our ability to focus. The gut has 200–600 million neurons and it communicates with us using various gut feelings, such as 'butterflies in our stomach' when we are excited or in love, or 'a knot in our stomach' when we are worried or anxious. We talk about 'spilling our guts' when we let our emotions out.

The relationship between our psyche and gut works both ways: diseases of the gut affect our minds and moods, and vice versa. Iain McGilchrist brings together results from various studies in his book *The Matter With Things* (2021), showing that the gut produces 95 per cent of the body's serotonin, a chemical that carries messages between nerve cells in the brain and the rest of the body. Serotonin is needed for the nerve cells and brain to function; and this hormone plays a key role in body functions like sleep, mood change, digestion, nausea, wound healing, bone health, blood clotting and sexual desire. Serotonin mediates satisfaction, happiness and optimism; and, conversely, its levels are reduced in depression.

Gut feelings are important signals that we can learn to understand with practice. Over time, you may find it easier to discern which gut reactions are related to food or hormones, and which are related to choices you are making. Our gut feelings will never be foolproof, but they can give us important clues.

CONNECT WITH YOUR GUT

This exercise is especially good if you are worried, stressed or anxious.

1. Take a few deep breaths and observe how your breathing moves your stomach.

- Listen to what your stomach is telling you it needs. Does it want extra-deep breaths? Or does it want a stretch?
- Notice if it is calm or anxious.
- Ask yourself questions and see if your stomach reacts to them.
- Your questions could be: How are you doing [your name]? Is [insert] the right choice for me at this point? Am I afraid of [insert]?

2. Lie on your back and take two or three deep breaths to settle into the position.

- Breathe in deeply, keep it in and on the count of four, breathe out until there's no more air to exhale; now suck in your stomach two or three times, and hold in your breath.
- When you can't hold it in any longer, let it out and fill your lungs with air again.
- Do this a few times.

The vagus nerve and two strands of the nervous system

Vagus nerve carries information from the brain to most of the body's major organs, slows everything down and allows self-regulation. It's the nerve that is associated with the parasympathetic system and emotions like love, joy and compassion.

DEEPAK CHOPRA

The vagus nerve is the longest cranial nerve in the body, connecting almost all our major organs, from the brain to the colon, including the learning centres in the brain. It comes from the Latin word *vagus*, meaning 'wandering', because it wanders widely, connecting the brainstem to every part of the body. This system controls specific bodily functions such as digestion, heart rate and immune system. These functions are involuntary, which means that we can't consciously control them.

The vagus nerve reminds us that the body is an interconnected whole and it plays an important role in our ability to self-regulate, calm down and be resilient. When the vagus nerve gets damaged, there will obviously be neck pain but other symptoms may include an increased heart rate, brain fog, excessively high or low blood pressure, gut problems, and issues with the voice or throat. So when we speak, shout, chant or sing, we activate the vagus nerve, which is one reason why those activities can be so cathartic and emotional.

The autonomic nervous system is divided into the sympathetic nervous system ('fight or flight') and the parasympathetic nervous system ('rest and digest'); this dual system maintains a balance within the body and does a good job of keeping us alive and functioning well. The parasympathetic system is a calm learning mode, while the sympathetic system is a stressed mode that helps protect us from danger.

The vagal nerves are the main nerves in the para-sympathetic system, which helps trigger a relaxation response in our body and is activated when the perceived danger or stress is over. Sometimes, however, our stress levels remain too high for too long and we need to mindfully help our nervous system to calm down. To help us activate and access our InnSæi, it is important to calm our minds, and find a balance between the two systems, with simple techniques such as grounding, meditation, mindfulness and breath work. Yoga, exercises and outdoor activities can also help us connect mind and body in order to embody InnSæi. Here are a few exercises you can do to activate your parasympathetic system.

BREATH WORK – BREATHING THROUGH YOUR DIAPHRAGM

- Place one hand on your stomach and the other hand on your chest.
- As you breathe in, feel your stomach expand, and when you exhale, your stomach should go back down. This is also known as 'belly breathing'.
- Exhale longer than you inhale. Try pursing your lips together to restrict the exhale, as if you are blowing up a balloon.
- Do this a few times and feel the calming effect it has on your system.

COLD WATER ON YOUR FACE AFTER EXERCISE

- Physical exercise causes an increase in sympathetic activity(the 'fight or flight' mode) and the stress response, resulting in a higher heart rate.
- Studies have found that immersing your face in cold water is a simple way to reactivate the parasympathetic system through the vagus nerve. This reduces your heart rate, calms you down and activates your immune system.
- Cold water on face (or body) is also effective in

a non-exercise environment in order to activate the vagus nerve.

'OM' CHANTING

- A great way to activate your vagus nerve is by chanting 'OM' over and over again.
- Feel how the sound vibrates inside you, from the belly and root of the vagus nerve up to the head.
- *Om* is a very simple sound with a complex meaning. It represents the union of mind, body and spirit, and it is often used in yoga, mantras and different faiths such as Hinduism and Buddhism. It helps to calm you and create a sense of inner peace.

Main keys to InnSæi:

* InnSæi means the *sea within*, to *see within*, and to *see from the inside out*.

* InnSæi is an embodied feeling. We centre ourselves and connect with InnSæi through the whole body. Listen and pay attention to how your body speaks to you and you to it.

* Silence the noise inside and outside your head in order to access InnSæi.

* The rational mind's chattering thoughts, stress, material or financial pressures can block the flow of InnSæi.

* InnSæi is timeless; it weaves ancient wisdom together with modern science and sees everything as interconnected.

* We all have InnSæi. It is our inner compass; it is up to us to tune into it and regularly update it.

* We are not our thoughts; we are the thinkers of our thoughts. When our connection to InnSæi is blurred, we doubt ourselves, and we become undecisive and less confident.

* We communicate beyond words, with our whole body, through energy fields and brainwaves.

* Practice, expertise and self-knowledge strengthen our InnSæi.

* Practise aligning with InnSæi. When we are aligned with InnSæi we intrinsically get how everything is interconnected and we connect more deeply with our own humanity.

* Self-awareness enables us to balance our energy and understand how to optimise our InnSæi. When we are losing ourselves in a situation, we find safety by bringing our mind back to our

body. We open up to our senses and notice how the world comes to us.

* Attention is the key to self-awareness, creativity and InnSæi. Pay attention to what you pay attention to, with your whole body, and jot it down in your journal. Don't judge what you pay attention to, only witness it.

Chapter 2

The Healing Power of InnSæi

Look at you, look around us, people unhappy, people disturbed, we are totally disconnected from the brain and the body. So many people live in their heads and they don't live with emotions, something must be deeply wrong.

MARINA ABRAMOVIĆ, PERFORMANCE ARTIST, SPEAKING IN
THE DOCUMENTARY FILM *INNSÆI – THE SEA WITHIN*

In my late twenties I hit a wall, lost direction and descended into darkness. The darkness forced me to connect *within*, as I had nowhere else to go. From there, I re-emerged a slightly different person and it has shaped my life ever since. My story – about losing hope in life, about my body caving in to alert me to my disconnection from InnSæi – is by no means unique. Many people, all over the world, have similar experiences.

We all have an innate need to belong, to find purpose and meaning in our lives. Within a period of roughly four years, I went from being aligned with my InnSæi, fearlessly navigating by it as my inner compass, to losing my connection with it and, in the process, my sense of direction, confidence, belonging and purpose. When I reconnected with my InnSæi, it was like coming home to myself, except that I was now even more conscious of being nurtured and guided by it. Emerging from this humbling journey brought deeper laughter, more tears and gratitude, and the courage to give myself permission to live life more fully than ever before. Rediscovering my link to InnSæi, and learning how to align to its rhythms, meant that the world inside and around me started to move and flow. I had begun the process of healing.

More often than not, the pain we feel is trying to tell us something about ourselves and the place we find ourselves in. This chapter is an invitation to explore the idea of allowing ourselves to grow through pain and why it is important to make space in our lives for melancholy and vulnerability, and ask hard questions about life, love and purpose.

From a young age, I dreamt about working on human rights with the Red Cross or the United Nations, in the hope of helping to make the world a better place. The 1990s was a defining decade for me – I was in my early twenties, I finished college and two university degrees and worked as a journalist on foreign news.

In 1993 I saw the film *In the Name of the Father*, a true story of four people falsely convicted of the 1974 Guildford pub bombing in Surrey, England, and it inspired me to sign up as a volunteer with Amnesty International. There was conflict in the former Yugoslavia at that time, and when I had to choose a subject for my undergraduate dissertation in social anthropology at the University of Iceland a few years later, I swung between wanting to explore how music reflects undercurrents in modern culture, and wanting to research civil disobedience during the wars in the former Yugoslavia. Both these ideas occurred to me because I tuned my antenna and paid attention to the world around me. The more I tried to put myself in the shoes of the people going through these wars, the more I wanted to know.

Mainstream media was telling a story about a religious and ethnic war between 'good guys' and 'bad guys', with terrible consequences for civilians who were being tortured, killed or forced to flee their homes. I had seen images of tanks, explosions and refugees, and I read reports by senior officials, mostly men, who were meeting to resolve the conflicts. But I intuitively knew that there was something I was missing from this narrative and I set out to ask my own questions. What would I do if I had been born into that situation? I wanted to know if people were trying to peacefully resist the wars or doing anything to promote peace. I ended up writing about informal and peaceful resistance during the wars in former Yugoslavia at both undergraduate and graduate level. As far as I could tell from my initial investigation, and consulting professors and professionals, this was a little researched topic at the time. In this way, my InnSæi was opening up a whole new world that I would otherwise not have discovered and leading me to people and places I had never imagined going to.

Empathy opens a window

I established contact with a diverse group of people through the internet, who generously helped me understand the story of informal resistance during the wars, telling me a story I could not find anywhere else. People resisted the wars peacefully, through radio and print media, human rights activism, film making, music and graphic art. They redesigned historic posters, like Uncle Sam's famous wartime call to recruit soldiers. Instead of the original message, 'I Want You! For U.S. Army', they wrote, 'I Want You – to Save Sarajevo', a Bosnian city that was under siege for three years.

People sent me their diaries and shared with me their calls for action and support from mainstream media and politicians in Europe and the US. I interviewed people from the former Yugoslavia, wider Europe, Russia and the US, through emails and phone calls, who had helped raise awareness of the situation. In 1991, one of my interviewees helped set up an online communications system across the republics to counter state-run war propaganda. As we know, there's massive power invested in controlling the flow of information and media at any given time, and history has taught us that information plays a key role in manufacturing narratives, including those on wars and polarisation. This communication system, designed to counter state-run propaganda by promoting dialogue and solidarity, was called ZaMir, which means 'for peace' in Serbo-Croatian. It was an email system that enabled people from the former Yugoslavia to organise support and logistics and correct false news across battle lines. My contact and one of its founders generously gave me access to five years of communications, from 1991 to 1995, which I saved on a bunch of floppy discs, read and analysed. By empathising with strangers and following my InnSæi into unknown territory, I had opened a window into a world which would otherwise have been invisible to me.

ZaMir was up and running about two years before the internet launched into the public domain, and almost ten years before social media started. Writing about this now, I wonder how different things might have been if the business models of social media today were truly about promoting dialogue and solidarity, instead of creating loneliness and polarisation, while putting all their efforts into 'hacking our minds' and capturing our attention.

As I was nearing the end of my BA thesis in late 1998, conflict was still raging in Kosovo, which was then in Serbia. An American professor I had sought advice from a few weeks earlier, sent me the email address of a woman called Igballe Rogova, one of Kosovo's most prominent human rights activists, so that I could interview her for my BA thesis. However, we decided against doing the interview, in case it put her in danger, given the full-blown conflict taking place in Kosovo at the time. But I later discovered how small the world is, and how it is shaped by where we direct our attention and the relationships we build, because a little less than three years later, in 2001, I had moved to Kosovo and was working alongside Igaballe Rogova, or Igo as we call her. And in 2004, when I went back to Kosovo for a short work trip, her computer screen saver was a picture of my newborn daughter Rán. Who could have imagined that, only four years earlier?

The ripple effects of wars

The war in Kosovo ended in June 1999 and the post-war reconstruction and peace-building started. In 2001 I became the programme manager for one of the UN agencies in Kosovo, which at the time was called UNIFEM. I was 27 years old, worked there for a year and that year felt like ten years packed into one. I soon discovered that wars do not end with peace agreements; they have ripple effects that spread through generations into the future.

Going to Kosovo was like walking into an open wound. I could see and smell the aftermath of conflict in the air, in people's eyes and physical expressions and the ruined houses and buildings. A collapsed white orthodox church lay like a broken bird by the road. A sports centre and people's homes, riddled with bullet holes, bore witness to the violence. There was rubbish everywhere, a rank smell in the air; stray dogs sniffing the ground, adjusting to street life after losing their homes and families. People who couldn't make eye contact, full of fear, anger, but mostly exhaustion and broken hearts.

The so-called 'abandoned children', conceived through violence or unrecognised love between people from opposite sides of the war, were left – on doorsteps and parking lots – to the mercy of God, strangers or monsters. At the hospital in Pristina, the capital of Kosovo, those friendless little souls lay in plastic cribs with cockroaches crawling over them, sour milk thick and dry on their cheeks. The Red Cross engaged a group of us to go and visit them after work. The aim was simply to show them kindness, to touch and hug them, because no one else would. Without that human touch, they would be less able to develop the emotional skills needed to experience intimacy and trust with other human beings.

War brings forth death and destruction and you can feel it, even if you haven't lived it. You pick it up with your senses. Most of it sneaks under the radar of your conscious mind and alerts your nervous system. It pops up in the form of nightmares so real that you think bugs are crawling over your body at night – you try to scream as loud as you can but no sound comes out.

In Kosovo, all I wanted was to make a difference for the victims of war, and contribute to a peaceful and democratic future; but I had no idea how to set personal boundaries, nor did I even understand why that was important. I believed that taking time for myself, to recharge my batteries, would be a sign of weakness.

Although I thought I knew how to deal with the trauma and sorrow that surrounded me, I was only closing myself off from these emotions, locking them inside my body, and continually pressuring myself to do better. My sleep deprivation grew, as did the nerve pain from slipped discs in my spine. Eventually I got so disconnected from myself that I was forced to think again.

While traveling from Kosovo to Kazakhstan, I spent a night at Frankfurt airport and, the morning before my second flight, I was in terrible pain and started to bleed.

I didn't think too much of it – just took some painkillers and continued my journey. It was only later that I realised I'd had a miscarriage. This should have been a wake-up call, but instead I kept ploughing on.

Whether I'd had a miscarriage because I'd been pushing myself too hard, or the pregnancy just wasn't meant to be, whatever the circumstances, this episode certainly showed how disconnected I had become from my own body and emotions. My way of coping was to put aside my physical and emotional health, thinking I just needed to be thick-skinned. Or perhaps I was so passionately consumed by my work that I didn't notice the disconnection from my soul.

A path back home

Before moving to Kosovo I had taken an international competitive exam in Reykjavík, Iceland, in the hope of becoming a public servant with the United Nations. This was a rare opportunity. If I succeeded, it meant I would spend my life serving the UN, working in different departments and regions of the world. While I was in Kosovo, I received a letter signed by the UN Secretary General, Kofi Annan, offering me a post starting at the UN Economic Commission for Europe in Geneva, Switzerland.

In summer 2002, I moved from Kosovo to Geneva, to

take up a permanent position at the United Nations, feeling excited at how fast my career seemed to be taking off. My office was in the Palais des Nations, in a graceful building with spacious gardens, gorgeous peacocks on the lawn, and a view of Mont Blanc that was as beautiful on the outside as it became stifling for me on the inside. Unfortunately, the hierarchy and bureaucracy in Geneva had a numbing effect; it was so different from the responsibility and leverage we'd had to make real changes in Kosovo. UNIFEM was still piloting its post-conflict reconstruction work during my time there, which gave us an active, entrepreneurial working environment, still a bit removed from the rigid administration structure of the UN . In Kosovo we were in direct contact with the people who relied on our support, while in the institutional environment in Geneva, at the UN Economic Commission for Europe covering 55 member states, I felt disconnected from the rest of the world. I began to feel I was serving a system, instead of the system serving the people and the planet.

I became frustrated and absent-minded, and started planning early retirement because I didn't have the courage to resign. Not feeling fulfilled at work didn't seem like a good enough reason to leave and I continued to dismiss my inner voice and InnSæi. In hindsight, I can see that my InnSæi was trying to get my attention through day-dreaming, small hunches and my remarks in some of the conversations I was having with friends and family. I was planning what to do when I retired after almost three decades. I envisaged myself in my late fifties – I would write and be a change-maker, focusing on enhancing people's creative agency and a sustainable future. It was during this time that my fiancé and I decided to start our own family. We had been together for about ten years, and before we knew it I was pregnant with our first child. At least my personal life seemed to be thriving and the future felt bright.

But if there is anything I learned at this point in my life, it is that we can take nothing for granted. The job I thought I'd always wanted, and worked hard to get, ended up making me feel stagnant and unfulfilled, and soon my relationship with the man I loved began to break down.

We decided to have our daughter in Iceland and, by the time she was born, things had changed for the worse, and our relationship was hanging by a thread. Separation seemed like the only way forward and I was heartbroken. Soon my maternity leave would end and so I started to organise my return to Geneva, this time as a single mother. I found a new flat and arranged childcare, but once all that had been organised, the question kept creeping up on me: *Is this what I really wanted to do?*

No one could answer this but me and, given the state I was in, it wasn't easy. I had been sleep-deprived for months, my nervous system was weak and tense and at one point, when a nurse asked me to take a deep breath, I literally couldn't – I just didn't have the energy. The back pains kept coming back and I was diagnosed with three slipped discs and told I might not be able to work full-time again. I found it hard to share my challenges with others and felt lost and alone. I was a mess.

Giving birth to my daughter taught me so much about my body and focused my attention on it in ways I had never conceived of before; I was in awe of its complexity, resilience and power to carry a beautiful soul and bring her into this world. The slipped discs in my spine, where much of my neurosystem is located, also kept my focus on my body until I truly realised I had to start from there. I learned to listen to it, to build physical and mental strength. I learned to prepare beautiful, healthy food, and eat more mindfully, and I started to feel how the body and mind are interrelated and can be mutually supportive.

To clear the way to the core of my soul and activate my InnSæi, I decided to keep a journal about what I was going through, write different kinds of sentences, and experiment with how they made me feel when I read the words on paper. I realised my InnSæi spoke to me most clearly through my stomach; and some sentences made it knot up, while others made it feel calmer. I did my best to let my emotions and thoughts out on the paper, trying not to judge my writing but to simply acknowledge and face whatever I was feeling.

I spent a lot of time outside, walking my daughter in a comfortable stroller, breathing in the fresh air by the coast where I lived or in the national park close by. I loved my daughter in a way I had never felt before, and caring for her gave me happiness. I could feel the healing and grounding power of nature and Iceland's strong winds clearing my thoughts, along with the cathartic process of journaling. I found I was able to think a bit more openly about my options, in a situation that had felt very tight and constraining. I gradually confided in a few close friends who supported me, and slowly the thoughts that had been swirling uncontrollably in my head, keeping me awake at night, gave way to a calmer, clearer headspace. One day, when I was walking on the coast where I lived, a question occurred to me: *Hrund, when you grow old, how do you want to look back on your life?*

And it came to me, like a short film, with scenes from my future life, showing a very different me. Suddenly I saw myself as a woman who was free to explore and speak her mind, had travelled the world and lived a fulfilling life. The sensation was so real, I could feel it in my body. This was the life I wanted. I knew what to do and the knowing brought a powerful inner stillness and peace. While most things in my life were still a mess, at that moment somehow it seemed that everything had fallen into place. A few days later, I resigned from my permanent position at the UN.

This was a leap of faith into the unknown. All I knew was that it was the right thing for me to do at that time. In the months that followed, I had physiotherapy; I sought advice from healers and wise people; I read everything I could find about the mind-body connection and creativity; and I learned how to piece myself back together, trust in life and flow a bit more. I learned to stop resisting things that were already changing and gained the courage I needed to face my fears.

One of the toughest things to deal with was the identity crisis that came with having left my permanent position at the UN, having no job title and no solid career plan. Who was I, without a job? How could I leave my dream job and a secure income? My career had taken off with a bang a few years earlier and was impressive by most people's standards, not least in view of the unique opportunities I had been given at such a young age. I felt as if I had fallen off a cliff, or a pedestal, and it took quite some time to rebuild my self-confidence.

I began to understand how difficult emotions were knotted up in my body, making my muscles and joints as stiff as rocks. My spine took time to get better; I was constantly in pain and it was often a real challenge simply to pick up my daughter to hold her in my arms.

I remember the day when I could reach down to touch my toes again, one and a half years after she was born. I started practising mindfulness, and different types of yoga and meditation, and I learned for the first time the value of preparing healthy food for simple meals that looked both colourful and beautiful.

I began to be more conscious of receiving support and kindness from others and to reward myself for small victories. I learned about the important balance between giving and receiving, doing and being, planning and creating. This was all an important part of showing myself more kindness and care. I started to laugh more, rest more, cry more and to love my imperfections instead of seeking perfection. I took the advice of wiser people and travelled back in time to reconnect with my inner child in me; I started drawing, painting and writing again. Reawakening my creativity turned out to be a crucial part of my healing process. I wrote short stories, a play, poems, a novel, project proposals, designed the university module I would have wanted to attend myself, and took on various consultancy assignments that helped me pay my bills. Some of the stuff I wrote got published or put on stage; some of the projects I designed turned into reality, while others were rejected. Gradually, difficult emotions were released from the muddy waters within and clarity emerged.

STEPS TO CONNECT WITHIN AND HEAL

- Sleep or rest whenever you can.
- Breathe deeply – and twice as long on the out-breath. Notice how this calms your nervous system.
- Work with and through your pain. Write and talk about it. Express it in any way that is constructive. If you resist or suppress it, it will persist.
- Spend time in nature, noticing textures, colours, smells and the behaviour of animals.
- Smile – and notice how this affects you and others.
- Experience how time expands and slows down when you are fully present in the moment.
- Journal every day to release emotions and thoughts and quiet your mind (see Chapter 4).
- Make your food with care, skill and love. Drink plenty of water.

LIFE THROUGH THE EYES – A FIVE-MINUTE MEDITATION

- Find a comfortable position, close your eyes and take deep breaths.
- Notice your breath breathe you.
- Imagine your eyes as beautiful embers.

- As you breathe in, feel your eyes sparkle with energy.
- As you breathe out, smile with your eyes.
- Repeat as often as you wish.

My friend, pain

This pain it is a glacier moving through you
And carving out deep valleys
And creating spectacular landscapes
And nourishing the ground
With precious minerals and other stuff

'GLACIER', SONG BY BIRGIR THORARINSSON AND JOHN GRANT,
LYRICS BY JOHN GRANT, FROM THE ALBUM *PALE GREEN GHOSTS*
(BELLA UNION, 2013)

Pain in the soul takes longer to heal than a broken leg. When we resist changes that are already in motion, or experiences that are hard to deal with, it doesn't make them go away; they get frozen inside us instead. Glaciers and pain bring great lessons about time: you never see the calving of ice in reverse; life never goes in reverse. Scientists call it 'the arrow of time'. It is important to keep moving, letting go and growing through pain. InnSæi, the sea within, implies constant movement and the logic of water. If it gets frozen or put into silos, it ceases to flow. Resisting pain and shutting down our emotions freezes the sea within. Showing our pain warmth and kind attention helps unleash difficult emotions and melt the ice inside us.

Pain is all around us – and perhaps in you at this very moment. What do we make of pain in all its varied forms? Do we numb it or do we allow ourselves to feel it and grow through it? We may give ourselves time to work through pain in stages, and that's fine. Difficult experiences tend to revisit us throughout our lives, in different forms, depending on the context and the work we've done to process and heal them.

As in John Grant's lyrics, pain moves through us with time, like a glacier that melts, nourishing us with different minerals and shaping our inner landscape in the process. People may be going through pain without us knowing; it doesn't always show on the outside. We can also be in pain and be happy at the same time. Life is complex. With time and attention, emotions transform, flow, mutate or evaporate like water, if we can forgive and let go. Gradually we heal.

Trauma is a big word – one that I used to avoid using. But I've come to accept that we all go through traumas in our lives, starting when we are born. 'The key to healing and growing through pain and trauma is to understand that the brain and body are designed to heal themselves,' says Dr Rebekah Granger-Ellis, an expert in neurowellbeing and neurobiology of learning, who has worked with some of the foremost business leaders and international organisations on shifting mindsets, healing trauma, and developing resilience in children, teens and adults. Trauma can be any adverse life experience, from neglect, bullying, rejection, loss of a loved one, to family dysfunction, hunger, poverty or violence. 'What the brain interprets and perceives as trauma, is trauma to the brain and body,' she explains but reminds us that 'we were born to regenerate, and that includes our brain and nervous system – we are remarkably neuroplastic'. We are our own healers in so many ways.

History is full of myths that teach us we can emerge from difficult experiences and be reborn as stronger leaders, more whole or wiser people. These myths are there for us to learn from. One of them is the story of Inanna, the Mesopotamian Goddess of Heaven and Earth, who goes to see her sister, Ereshkigal, who lives in the underworld and is the Goddess of Death. Ereshkigal represents Inanna's shadow side, her own underworld and imperfections. Here's a short version of the myth:

One day Inanna learns that Ereshkigal's husband has died, and she wishes to attend his funeral. Inanna's trusted adviser, Ninshubur, begs her not to go because she fears for her life. But Inanna insists; she needs to go and mourn with her sister and tells Ninshubur to send help if she does not return in three days. Before she departs on her journey, Inanna puts on her full queenly regalia and heads down to the underworld alone, where her sister reigns.

On her way down to the underworld, Inanna has to enter a few gates and at each of them she is forced to give up some of her garments and jewellery, which symbolise her status, identity and power. At each gate, another layer of her identity is peeled off: her crown, necklace and belt, symbolising her divinity, voice and willpower; her ornamented staff and cloak, emblems of authority and sovereignty. All these trappings are taken from her, until she arrives in the underworld, completely naked and vulnerable. Her ego is damaged and no sister's warm welcome awaits her. Instead, Ereshkigal receives her by announcing that the price of coming to the underworld is death. She then kills her sister Inanna and hangs her on a meat hook to rot.

*After three days and three nights, Inanna has not
returned and her trusted adviser, Ninshubur, gets
help from Enki, the God of Wisdom and Water.
He creates two tiny beings from the dirt under
his fingernails. These two creatures have only
one skill, and that is empathy. They fly so fast
that the gatekeepers don't even see them. When
they arrive in the underworld, they see Inanna
hanging naked from a hook and her sister writhing
in pain on the floor. The two tiny beings go over
to Ereshkigal to show her empathy and help her
heal. When she feels better, she thanks them and
asks if there is anything she can do for them. The
two tiny beings ask for the body of Inanna and
so Ereshkigal gives them the body and all of her
belongings. They take her above the ground and
back to heaven, and revive her. She lives to reign
again, wiser than before.*

Inanna's journey down to the underworld is about facing
our shadow sides, shedding our skin and growing through
pain. 'You cannot grow a lotus without mud,' said the
Zen Buddhist master Thich Nhat Hanh, and the deeper
the pain we go through, the greater our ability to savour
beauty and happiness. Inanna was reborn after facing her
own underworld, represented by her sister, Ereshkigal.

Inanna's myth teaches us that material wealth and the external trappings of status are fleeting; and it is only when we shed our skin, feathers, ego or decoration that we can come home to ourselves. The experience can range from moments of embarrassment or humiliation to feeling great pain or fear. We tend to hide our vulnerabilities from the outside world and think we need to perform, show up or look as if all is well, perhaps sometimes even fake perfection. That is a lot of pressure to put on ourselves.

InnSæi connects us to ourselves, other people and the world around us. Facing our shadows and darkest moments is an important part of acknowledging who we are and what we are capable of. Inanna's myth reminds us that it is sometimes our most difficult life experiences that bring forth our greatest strength and sense of purpose. You may already have discovered this in yourself or the people around you. Here are three examples of such people: the explorer Mark Pollock, Dr Rebekah Granger-Ellis and the Nobel Peace Prize Laureate Wangari Maathai.

My friend Mark Pollock is a warm, fun and smart explorer from Ireland. I first met Mark in 2014 at Oxford University and remember being deeply touched by his radiant smile and matter-of-fact energy when he told me his mission is to find a cure for paralysis in our life-time. I had never met anyone with such a bold goal before.

Mark Pollock is an explorer, speaker and a leadership

coach. When Mark was five, he lost the sight of his right eye and was forced during the remainder of his childhood to avoid contact sports to preserve the vision in his left eye; nevertheless he became an avid and competitive rower. Aged 22 he lost the sight of his left eye and became blind. Driven as he is, Mark Pollock transformed his blindness into a strength and became the first blind person to race to the South Pole. He competed in some of the world's most difficult races, completing six marathons in seven days in the Gobi desert, as well as a host of other endurance events. When he was 34 years old, three years before I met him, Mark was left paralysed after falling from a third-storey window. Lying in the hospital right after the accident Mark wondered if life was worth carrying on with all of the challenges that he was now facing. For the first few months, the question was related to simply getting up in the morning, getting washed and dressed, being in his wheelchair, going to the rehab gym, the effort to try to just exist in the world. 'In the aftermath of paralysis, I certainly asked myself the question is it worth it? The answer was always the same – that it was and is worth carrying on,' he explains.

Mark's experience shaped the projects that he focused on, switching from endurance racing to offering himself up as a human guineapig in research labs. Over a ten-year period, scientists and tech innovators tested what would happen if they combined wearable exoskeletons that would allow him to stand and walk with a spinal stimulator on his lower back to promote voluntary movement. The impact was dramatic, but Mark saw that the work was too fragmented and switched his 'efforts to creating the condition for collaboration amongst scientists, technologists, investors and philanthropists to help get the experimental technology commercialised.' The collaboration fed into the conversations that eventually led to a company called Onward being formed. As Mark said: 'My job wasn't to be the scientist or to have the money or to form any of the companies. However, I could bring what I had learned about working with people under pressure as an endurance athlete to the projects.' Onward is a start-up company that was founded towards this end, and when Mark and I spoke, they had just raised 100 million USD. 'I hope companies like Onward will start to become the norm, rather than the exception, and will speed up progress towards finding a cure for paralysis in our lifetime,' Mark explained. The Onward Arc Therapy is a targeted, programmed stimulation of the spinal cord, aimed to enable people with spinal cord injury to move again.

We are our own healers

Mark turned his hardest experiences into his strength and sense of purpose, as we will continue to explore in Chapters 3 and 5. His personal challenges, and the setbacks from these, shaped him as the person and into the leader he now is.

Dr Rebekah Granger-Ellis is also someone who has turned her most difficult life experiences into her vocation and mission in life. At age 33, a lifetime of suppressed trauma had stretched her physical and mental boundaries to a breaking point and her 'body started to break down, even at the most basic cellular level,' she explains. 'Mysterious symptoms began appearing and stacking on, one after another.' Her hair began falling out by the handful, peculiar rashes appeared all over her body; she would fall asleep while lecturing or driving from chronic fatigue, and obstructive sleep apnoea was followed by uncontrollable weight loss, intensive bleeding and early menopause. After two years of being referred from one doctor to another, she was diagnosed with 23 different conditions. At some point she was taking 70 different pills, a concoction of prescription pills and vitamins each day, and wasn't getting any better. By 35, she'd had a hysterectomy, lumpectomies in her breasts and legs, and numerous stays in the hospital for takotsubo cardiomyopathy and transient ischemic attacks. Her kidneys and liver were not functioning properly and her hormones or thyroid were dysregulated. 'I was diagnosed with severe anxiety because at this stage you feel everything is falling apart and it had worsened to the point where I was losing memory and cognitive functioning. I was writing and lecturing but I couldn't even remember certain words. I would confuse the word "blue" with "a table", for example. I would hear myself say it, but it wasn't what I thought in my mind. I was having so much disconnection neurologically.' It was at this point, a neurologist told her that, if left unadressed, she only had two or three years left to live.

In a desperate search for healing and understanding about what was happening to her health, Dr Rebekah plunged into extensive research herself and discovered that she needed to become her own healer. 'It was such a wake-up call,' she recalls, 'that you have to be your own advocate and healer because no one has the holistic view of your brain and body other than you.' Dr Rebekah was fortunate enough to find a neurologist who unlocked this realisation. After a day in a neurology diagnostic lab, running the full assessment battery, the doctor concluded that she had no memory dysfunction. Instead, in the spirit of holistic healing, he asked her to tell him her life's story, from beginning to the end.

Rebekah began sharing her personal story and releasing with it all the difficult memories and emotions that had been trapped inside her body over the years. 'I did a lot of crying that day, and I realised that I had become so numb that I had stopped crying years ago. This was such an overwhelming release of stored trauma.' Rebekah's story is marked with childhood sexual abuse, a toxic and abusive marriage, and chronic stress from working with trauma populations. Through her personal relationships and passion for her challenging work, she had spent her life internalising the trauma and stories of others. She had not only shown others empathy, but also took on herself other people's pain, with the sincere belief that she could love someone enough that they would heal. Like me during my time in Kosovo, she did not know how to set boundaries or limitations on herself. The neurologist explained to her cortisol neurotoxicity, stress-induced neurodegeneration, and brain and body budgeting, and he emphasised how critical it is to detox our minds and bodies. He advised her to seek therapy to heal from past traumas and to clear her life of unhealthy relationships and toxic stress. 'You need to get help and you need to get safe, otherwise at this rate, you will probably die in two or three years,' he concluded.

More than ten years had passed since she transformed her life, and since then she has finished her post-doctorate degree in neurobiology and neuroscience of learning, merging all that she'd learned in order to help people heal from trauma and chronic stress and to understand the body and brain systems holistically. Today, Dr Rebekah Granger-Ellis is an award-winning researcher and practitioner who has spent the last 20 years pioneering interventions for policy reforms and systems change with an extensive global network of leading minds. In partnership with government ministry and leading organisations and UNICEF and the World Bank, she has worked with survivors of trauma in different parts of the world, such as orphans in Guatemala, survivors of Hurricane Katrina in the US and the earthquakes in Turkey, and generations in the Western Balkans affected by the traumas brought by the wars.

Mark Pollock and Dr Rebekah Granger-Ellis not only went through physical and mental shocks that brought them to their knees; they managed to emerge from them stronger and more passionate about their leadership and purpose in life. But not everyone manages to stand up from falling down. Why are some people very resilient and others much less so and have a harder time healing themselves? Rebekah's face lights up when I ask her, it is so obvious we are talking about things she is passionate about. She spent eight years researching neuroscience of adaptability and adverse experiences, and in addition to her own research and two others she refers to (see Notes), she cites a King's College London meta-analysis, which includes over 85 years of research in resilience, and she explains the three main characteristics of what she calls 'resilient and adaptively intelligent individuals'.

Three main characteristics of resilient individuals

1. Psychologically safe, trusted connection

* A one-on-one connection with a deeply trusted person, someone who you can always go to for help, advice and a different perspective.

* This 'positive social support' can even overcome environmental and genetic vulnerabilities in increasing resilience.

2. A sense of humour

* The active coping strategy of humour and extroversion, the ability to not take yourself or life overly seriously.

* Laughing stimulates the vagus nerve and activates the parasympathetic nervous system, which helps maintain a balanced and healthy body budget and release dopamine, serotonin and oxytocin, creating a more positive and optimistic outlook.

3. Propensity to express positive emotions in relation to negative events

* An ability to see a hard experience through a

different lens, seeing that harm can be a gift for transformation, enables individuals to control their anxiety and fears.

* The ability to cognitively reframe, to say: 'That does not define me, I choose it as a gift to transform my purpose. I define myself on my own terms, and I change the world because of it.'

Sometimes life tests us to such an extent that the only way out is in. As I went through my life-changing experience, I remember feeling I was fighting for my life. I was genuinely afraid that I would not find my ground, hope or spark ever again. Every person on the planet will have to endure traumas, and challenging experiences that show up in different sizes and shapes, from our own birth, losing a loved one, major illness, conflict, neglect to divorce or professional failure. Throughout the centuries, humans have crafted myths and stories about how pain and difficult times can help us grow by coming home to ourselves. We can metaphorically or literally come close to death and experience rebirth. Major changes, whether forced upon us or self-initiated, can help us reinvent ourselves beautifully on our life's journeys, as long as we are aligned with InnSæi.

Trees and people with strong roots

The third story I want to share with you could just as well be a myth. It is, however, a true story about how grounding ourselves deeply in Mother Earth, and in our own souls, enables us to endure and grow through challenging times. It is the story of Wangari Maathai, who received the Nobel Peace Prize for the simple act of planting trees.

In *Unbowed: A memoir* (2006), Wangari Maathai recounts her extraordinary journey from her childhood in rural Kenya to the world stage. When her grandparents were growing up in the highlands in Kenya, they had four seasons a year and there was food for all its people. But colonialism, and unsustainable management of their natural resources, seriously disrupted their lives, the natural cycles of the ecosystem, causing social instability and desertification.

The trees traditionally grown in Kenya, like the fig tree, grew slowly and had strong roots that extended deep into the earth, breaking through rocks to reach fresh water deep in the ground, which then made its way along their roots up to the surface and kept the ecosystem hydrated and flourishing. However, in colonial times, local trees were replaced with new trees that grew faster, and could therefore be chopped down faster, shipped and sold to Europe. The new trees had weaker roots and were unable to help the water flow to the surface. This soon led to desertification and deterioration of the ecosystem. With colonialism came Christianity, the belief in one God in the sky, which replaced previous beliefs that had tied people closely to the land where they lived.

Wangari Maathai was the first woman in East and Central Africa to earn a doctorate degree; and when she returned to Kenya, she made it her mission to re-establish the vital relationship her people had with the earth and to revive its natural ecosystems. She founded the Green Belt Movement in 1977 and began a vital poor people's environmental movement, focused on the empowerment of women, that soon spread across Africa. She persevered through run-ins with the Kenyan government and personal losses. She was jailed and beaten on numerous occasions but continued to fight to save Kenya's forests and to restore democracy in her country. We decided to dedicate our documentary film *InnSæi – The Sea Within* to Wangari Maathai, because her focus on planting trees with strong roots created ripple effects, in the shape of social and political changes in her home country. In our view, her work was a beautiful example of the magic of InnSæi – when we attend to our own invisible roots, which go deep into our souls and Mother Earth, we can enable both ecosystems and individuals to thrive.

Projection of the inside and outside world

It is very possible to go through life like a zombie, a shadow of the person and soul that lies dormant inside you. You routinely do your work and fulfil your obligations; you meet friends and have a laugh but your laughter doesn't come from deep within; you cannot remember the last time you cried; moments of intimacy are rare if they exist at all; and you haven't felt a sense of awe and amazement for a long time. It is as if your body's cells are alive and doing their job, but they aren't lit up and beaming with life.

Facing my fears, befriending my pain and letting go of control and unhelpful beliefs, was a crucial part of my healing, rebirth and writing this book. During my worst moments, I felt trapped, both in the 'place' I was in and inside my own body. I had taken for granted my health, career, relationship and related future plans, almost seeing all this as the solid ground I stood on. When things started disintegrating, I kept ploughing on, but my body was signalling that not all was well. While I was experiencing disconnection on all these fronts, my greatest sense of disconnection was with my own soul. I knew I still had a strong sense of security and alignment somewhere inside me, and I set out to rediscover my inner compass.

When I resigned from what had been my 'dream job'

at the UN, it was not because I fleetingly felt lost in life or because I had become a mother, and possibly a single mother. It was because I felt that my own sense of disconnection from my InnSæi was reflected in what I saw in the world around me. It was as if a mirror was being held up, showing me and the system I worked within, and the image was fragmented, spiritless and incoherent. I had been learning how to navigate and serve a system, instead of working in a system that served and was in close contact with people and the planet. This was why I felt so disconnected, and I didn't believe it was the right way forward. From this point onwards, I decided that my work would revolve around finding a balance between our inner and outer worlds, and making room for aspects of life that are humane, creative and unquantifiable. I felt we had mistaken the map for the territory. We were focused on navigating with a map that showed the world as quantifiable and easily boxed-in, but we had lost sight of the territory, which is the magnificent, dynamic, ever-changing, animate and complex web of life.

I wanted to emerge from this siloed, lifeless system and send my roots in(to) the soil of the animate, living world, like Wangari Maathai's fig trees, to reconnect within, to people and the world around me. I wanted to be present, brave and generous in spirit. I could sense the prospect of all the cells in my body lighting up, shining like bioluminescent particles in the sea within, something that was invisible but fully embodied. My inner centre of gravity was shifting.

The idea of success and moving up a career ladder started to have quite a different meaning for me. I discovered that life wasn't about status, salaries or labels and my own worth did not come from material things, like medals, crowns or cloaks. What mattered most was to feel a deep sense of alignment from which all else unfolds. This became my core measure of success. I also wanted to have the courage to embrace my most vulnerable self in order to become my strongest self. I am still learning.

Pain brought me into my body and 'home to myself'. My InnSæi had been activated and I gained the confidence and sense of security that it brought. The more we are connected to the *sea within*, the more we are able to thrive, regenerate and sense our interconnectedness to the planet and people.

How we choose to train ourselves in seeing, sensing, living and co-creating our systems, processes and cultures will define the future of our lives on this planet. It is important that we activate our InnSæi in an ethical way in order to create the ripple effects that can bring about the world we dream of inhabiting. The Earth has planetary boundaries that define the limits of her ability to regenerate her energy. When we cross these planetary boundaries with excessive use of resources or the use of destructive chemicals, the Earth loses her ability to renew her complex ecosystems. We also need to acknowledge our own boundaries, and make sure we and others do not cross them, if we are to thrive. If all the change-makers, caretakers, innovators, entrepreneurs, creative thinkers and ecopreneurs out there stay aligned with their InnSæi, it will help all of us to be present and thrive in the turbulent times that lie ahead.

Main keys to InnSæi:

* The way through pain is to 'see it', own it and allow it to go through you.

* Pain speaks to us and it is important that we listen in order to heal.

* We are our own healers.

* Pain can get stored in our bodies and block our connection to InnSæi.

* When we attend to the pain, it can bring us home to ourselves and into our bodies.

* Put pain in motion by journaling about what you are going through, and confiding in someone you trust. Make sure you drink enough water, create, express yourself, stretch your body, release tensions in your body. All this will help you heal.

* Allow time for this work; don't force the process.

* InnSæi links your mind and body to your inner self. Disconnection from within can cause the body to collapse. Learn to listen to your InnSæi.

* InnSæi helps us put ourselves in other people's shoes. The spotlight of our attention takes us places and shapes our lives.

* Like the planet Earth, we have boundaries to protect us so that we can regenerate ourselves and stay aligned to InnSæi.

* Connecting deep within ourselves, and the Earth, enables us and ecosystems to flourish.

Chapter 3

The Sea Within

Understand and align with your InnSaei

When everything is connected to everything else, for better or for worse, everything matters.

BRUCE MAU, DESIGNER AND EDUCATOR

The world we live in is complex, volatile, fast-changing and non-linear. It is increasingly borderless when it comes to things like travel, finding your tribe, knowledge accumulation, climate change and technology. Everything is interconnected in a system where a small change in one place can cause an unforeseeable impact in another. A butterfly flaps its wings in Texas and causes a cyclone in Brazil. The fast-melting North Arctic ice causes sea levels on the Earth to rise so that hundreds of millions of people in other parts of the planet are forced to flee and relocate;

and capital cities by coasts are literally being moved to higher ground.

Metaphorically speaking, the world we live in is very much like the ocean. It is in constant motion, and the ever-changing, unpredictable directions of tides and waves challenge us to be conscious of where we go and how we get there. Living in this vast and complex world can feel like being alone on the ocean, with no land in sight. Rule number one is to keep your head up so you don't drown. Rule number two is to determine which direction to swim in. Now that's a harder one.

The ocean of consciousness

The ocean is the living heart and lungs of our home, planet Earth, and the oldest metaphor for consciousness. It covers about two-thirds of the surface of the Earth, provides us with healthy air to breathe and water to drink, to name just a few of the ways it helps us live. Now think about the *sea within*, how it behaves with its flow and ebb, its fluctuations between stillness and fury, cycles and stifled motion, its deepest calm and shallowest oscillations.

When the high winds or stormy weather of stress, fear and anxiety buffet us, they stir our minds, sometimes uncontrollably, just as howling gales or rainstorms do to the surface of the ocean. Yet, much like our minds, the bottom of the ocean is always the calmest part. To get there takes practice and self-control. When we meditate, mindfully breathing slowly and deeply, we reach the deepest calms, inner peace, clarity of mind and the strongest connection to our InnSæi.

All life on Earth emerged from deep in the ocean billions of years ago. Consciousness is so integral to our inner workings and is so natural to us, that we could easily go through life without giving it much thought. In many ways, it *is* life. This vast, intangible, invisible ocean of consciousness stretches way beyond the limits of our imagination. An imagined stone is thrown into it and creates ripple effects that we are mostly unaware of but which are likely to emerge later on, in the form of ideas, sentiments, dreams, reactions, decisions or 'aha' moments. The sea within us interacts constantly with the world around us so that it becomes unclear where I end, and you begin. Some say that there is a universal consciousness, of which human beings are an expression, in the same way that waves are an expression of the ocean on planet Earth. This would mean that we are waves on the ocean of consciousness. We are a part of it, and it is a part of us. Beautiful, right?

Imagine that you are standing on a beach, facing the ocean, the sea breeze on your face and hair, and as you smell and taste the sea on your lips you allow the sound of the waves to become one with your breath. You breathe in as the waves break on the beach and breathe out as they retreat. The deeper your breaths, the calmer your mind, and the more connected you become with yourself, other people and the world around you. This is energy in motion; the waves transmit energy within the ocean, just as your breath does within your being. As you look further towards the horizon you see the vast ocean, a seemingly endless body of water.

TEN-MINUTE MEDITATION
- **Find a comfortable position.**
- **Close your eyes.**
- **Visualise waves coming to and from the shore and hear the rhythmic sound they make.**
- **Breathe the waves in as they come to the shore; breathe them out as they go out to sea again.**
- **Feel the sea within you.**

I see you

We all long to be seen by others in a way that, for a start, recognises that we exist in the world, but also our contribution to life, our feelings and experiences, our needs and talents. When we are seen by others, it puts our energy in motion and strengthens us. That sense of belonging is crucial to our well-being, and it can give us a sense of purpose and meaning. Conversely, a loss of belonging can cause stress, decreased well-being, anger and depression.

To be seen by others and to be able to see others is part of the ecosystem of life – the feeling of being alive. It is how we light each other up and thrive. We are social animals. The way our civilisation has evolved is through storytelling and social interactions based on the stories we tell and believe are true. Communicating to another person that you actually *see* them, and feeling that you are seen by them, is not only done through words or sentences. Communications and signalling go way beyond the spoken and written word. It also takes place through body language and the interaction of invisible brainwaves that connect and synchronise between people's brains.

One of the most memorable and effective examples of this invisible, subtle communication between human beings was Marina Abramović's performance art piece, *The Artist is Present*, at the Museum of Modern Art (MoMA) in New York in 2010. In the performance, guests were invited to take a seat opposite Marina, one by one, and make long and deep eye contact with her. After three months and roughly 700 hours of sitting still on a hard wooden stool, communicating with people through the eyes, Marina's exhibition broke visitors' records in MoMA, one of the world's most popular art galleries. People waited in line; they even slept outside the museum to get a chance to be seen by her. By looking deeply into the 'soul's mirror' of complete strangers, Marina was able to express to them they were truly *seen* by her. 'The performance is really about presence,' Marina explained.

When we interviewed Marina in her star-shaped house outside New York for our documentary film *InnSæi – the Sea Within*, she talked about disconnection between people's hearts and heads:

> People today are disconnected because they live in their heads most of the time and not with their emotions... My function was to be 100 per cent present for them. To achieve that, the pattern of breathing is very important. You know, every time you breathe faster your concentration is less, but if you breathe rhythmically and slowly you can achieve that kind of state of mind of the moment which enables you to connect with the person in front of you. This is how you can make non-verbal communication possible.

Marina found that many of the visitors had 'tremendous pain' during the intense moments she and they shared, facing each other in the middle of the crowded museum.

'They project on me and I can feel their pain. And I was just the mirror, you know.'

The important part of the performance for Marina is to make us more aware that we are always busy. We never give ourselves the time to just sit on a chair and do nothing. But, she explains, 'in the moment you finally come and sit in front of me you are watched by the other people, you are filmed and watched by me, you have nowhere to escape. Nowhere, except into yourself, and when that happens, that connection clicks, then you really start being with your own self, which we actually avoid ... all our lives.'

She elaborated further: 'I think one of the successes of this piece was because it was not verbal. It was not about explaining emotion, it was about feeling them directly.' Because art is about expression, it has the potential to deeply affect and move people. It becomes infused with spirit, as well as matter. Imagine seeing a famous pianist on stage playing a piece with perfect technique but no passion or expression. Then imagine the pianist playing the same piece with the same technical skill but now with full emotional expression, with heart, gut and head in a perfect state of flow. The performance changes and it moves you – it has stirred the *sea within*.

When this happens, we witness the alchemy that takes place when people put their spirit and feelings into matter. Regardless of our job or vocation, every single one of us can inspire. We can either be generous in spirit or hide our souls from others. We can be connected to, or disconnected from, ourselves and other people. Marina decided to connect and be generous in spirit. That act of generosity put energy in motion and has moved thousands of people around the world, who continue to set up performances in her spirit, where strangers sit opposite each other and communicate through their eyes.

Spotlighting

Marina shifted our focused attention to the periphery of conventional human interaction and communication. Following her work, American and Russian scientists did research on Marina's brain where she repeated the act and sat in front of strangers and looked them in the eyes. Both had a scan on their heads, so-called electroencephalography (EEG), which monitored the brainwave activity and projected it on a screen above them. The screen showed how the brainwaves connected and communicated in thin air. When we interact with people on a given task, brain synchronicity takes place. The boundary between people's minds blurs and this can also happen between strangers in the same room. When we spend considerable time, or even live, together, our brains begin to synchronise, to the extent that we may begin to form similar thoughts and opinions.

The author and psychiatrist Iain McGilchrist has written extensively on the complex workings of the human brain and consciousness. Consciousness in the largest sense is commonly divided into the conscious (that of which we are aware of being aware) and unconscious (that of which we are unaware of being aware) – and only a small fraction of our mind is conscious. When we learn something new or need to solve a problem, we use our focused minds. But when things become familiar, like cycling, they sink into our unconscious where we no longer pay focused attention to them. Familiarity can trick us into zombie-like or numbed existence, where we no longer pay attention to what we are doing or seeing, the subtle cues and nuances that could enrich our lives and illuminate our presence. Iain explains that our intuition is our gateway to the unconscious minds and that if we would cut it out, we would be cutting out most of what we know, because very little of our mental processes are conscious – in fact, around 99 per cent of them are not conscious at all. 'Our intuition acts to alert us to things that our rather slow conscious mind may not be aware of,' he explained in the film *InnSæi*. Imagine your mobile phone showing one to five per cent charge? This is how little we are consciously aware of all that goes on around us and the inner workings of our minds.

It is important to remember that the conscious and

unconscious are not separate entities, but one big whole. Iain McGilchrist uses the image of a spotlight to explain this to help us understand the different ways we can chose to direct our attention. Imagine you are in the theatre and the wide and grand stage in front of you is pitch dark. A spotlight is suddenly turned on from the high ceiling and lights up one small part of the stage. The spotlight you see represents your conscious and focused mind. The rest of the stage is enormous, a bit like the ocean, with no hard edges. If you move the spotlight around you can give the edges of your focused mind more attention. For this we rely on our whole embodied being – head, heart, gut, hand and all our senses. In spite of it being intangible and hard to pin down, the unconscious is the most important and extensive part of our experience. In it, we discriminate, reason, analyse, find beauty, process challenges, solve problems, imagine possibilities, fall in love and so on, without being fully aware of it. It underlies everything else and if we want to, we can get to know it better and be better connected to it. When we attend to the world by moving our spotlight around by being with our senses, emotions and full body, exploring what is on the periphery of our focused and deliberate minds, we are more able to find balance between our intuition and reason, we are more able to be present.

HOW TO RE-ENGAGE YOUR CONSCIOUSNESS

- When you find yourself in a very familiar place (perhaps sitting in a meeting room, on the bus, or dining with your family or friends), pay attention to the things that are going on around you that you do not usually pay attention to. Notice how the people around you use their hands, the sounds they make in the space, the colours, movements, what each person says.
- Have a conversation with a stranger, listen actively to what they are saying and try to understand where they are coming from, without judgement.
- Take a detour from what you are used to doing. Walk an extra block, shop in a different neighbourhood that is very different from yours, listen to a radio station that's 'so not you', pay attention to everything that is green in a single day.

CALM THE SEA WITHIN FOR CLARITY

The word *emotion* originally meant 'to stir, move or agitate'. Let your emotions stir, move and agitate you, but don't let them drown you. Don't be the sea – navigate it.

- Find a comfortable position. Take a few deep breaths, release all tension and worries. Notice how this relaxes your body.
- Imagine the inside of your mind is spacious and white. You are able to walk into it and, as you do that, you look around to find a place to sit in.
- As you find your place, you look around and see your thoughts moving in circles around you, like pictures or short videos. All your thoughts and worries are flying around this white space inside your head.
- Mindfully watch them move around, acknowledge them, and then give them permission to leave your headspace. Do this until you can see in your mind and feel in your body that the white spacious area in your head is empty, peaceful and still.

Lit up by life

There's a good reason why Earth is often called 'the blue planet'. Almost all the world's water is found in the ocean and the ocean covers about 70 per cent of Earth's surface. Similarly, our human bodies largely consist of water and can only go two or three days without it. When we are born, we are about 75–80 per cent water, and this decreases proportionally as we grow older. When we die, the proportion of water in our bodies has gone down to 40–50 per cent. This is how fundamental water is to our energy and existence.

Furthermore, and partly through a complex interplay orchestrated between the sun, the moon and the tapestry of tiny little creatures that enable whole ecosystems to thrive, the ocean produces 50–80 per cent of the oxygen on Earth. That means that up to four out of five breaths you and I are taking at this very moment come from the sea. Imagine that! Our InnSæi functions with a similar purpose, guiding us to make decisions and ensuring our survival.

The main drivers of this amazing production of the life-giving oxygen on our planet are microscopic, drifting plants called phytoplankton or microalgae. They are mostly invisible to the naked eye, but with the help of a microscope we can see their beautiful shapes and forms, with the tiniest details and functional patterns. They truly are a work of art.

The surface layer of the world's ocean is teeming with these photosynthetic plankton that produce more oxygen than the largest redwoods, according to the National Oceanic and Atmospheric Administration. Despite amounting to only about 1 per cent of the global plant biomass, phytoplankton or microalgae account for at least half the oxygen production in our atmosphere. One species of bacteria, Prochlorococcus, is the smallest photosynthetic organism on Earth. This tiny bacterium produces up to 20 per cent of all the oxygen in the global biosphere, a higher per centage than all tropical rainforests combined.

All this goes to show that size really doesn't matter, and in a community of like-minded creatures we can light up the world with our purpose. When night falls, some of these marine organisms start to glow in the dark. If you haven't seen it, imagine you are looking over the surface of the ocean: you hear and see it moving rhythmically in the night, lit up by thousands of tiny lights. This is called bioluminescence, *bios* meaning 'life' and *lumen* meaning 'light'; they are lit up by life.

Like trees and other plants on land, phytoplankton have green-coloured chlorophyll which enables them to capture sunlight, photosynthesise and turn sunlight into energy. They also consume carbon dioxide (which in excessive doses creates pollution), and they release oxygen. What an incredibly purposeful life they lead!

Metaphorically speaking, I like to think that we humans also photosynthesise. A nice walk in the sun can energise us; the sun is vital to our existence, providing the vitamin D we need for healthy bones and a healthy immune system, which increases our well-being. Also, the more we can metaphorically absorb light – such as beauty, awe and positive energy – into our lives, the more energy we have and the more we can thrive and care as human beings.

The light in our lives increases when we are *seen* by the people we love and we can be generous in spirit towards others. You know that feeling – when you are all lit up, when you have that sparkle in your eyes, you look radiant or, better yet, you're on fire! We tell our loved ones to stay on the sunny side of life or thank them for being warriors of light when they bring positivity and love into our lives. And when life tests us to the limits and our energy is low, our light dims, and people may tell us 'there is light at the end of the tunnel'. At moments like these, it is good to remember that we are never alone, no matter how small and insignificant we may feel. We can light up our cells by mindfully visualising the waves in the ocean and taking deep breaths in and out. We stir up our *sea within* and help it flow, and stay dynamic, healthy, creative and vigorous. We can imagine our cells glowing in the dark, inside our bodies, much like phytoplankton riding the waves, and this makes us feel energised.

Without nature's ability to control the balance between carbon dioxide and oxygen in the atmosphere, we would not have enjoyed 10,000 years of stability in Earth's weather and ecosystems. Without a healthy balance between deep breaths in and out, between our intuitive and rational minds, the movement in our *sea within* is blocked. We need this balance to create energy, to emit light, to 'photosynthesise'.

WATER EXERCISE

- Listen to the sounds of water. You can listen online to meditative sounds of water, or go and sit by a fountain, river, stream or waterfall. Mindfully listen for a few minutes. Then imagine the sound is inside you.
- At home, find a comfortable position, close your eyes and take a few deep breaths to calm your mind.
- Imagine you are walking in a beautiful, green garden. You see a pond and walk up to it. Sit by the pond and watch your reflection in it. Is the water still or does it have ripples? Is your face clear or blurry?
- Through your mindful deep breaths, notice how the water gets stiller until it reflects you clearly, like a mirror image. Smile.

Flow

Be like water, my friend, making its way
through cracks. If nothing within you stays rigid,
outward things will disclose themselves.
BRUCE LEE, FROM SHANNON LEE, *BE WATER, MY FRIEND* (2020)

The more our *sea within* is circulating and flowing, the more the world will open up to us. The more we stop trying to control the things that are out of our hands, and trust the ocean of life, the more resilient and lighter we will be. The *sea within* sums up the borderless nature of our inner world, the universe inside every single one of us. It is a world that goes beyond words, a world of vision, feelings and imagination.

The *sea within* is constantly moving and making new connections out of the millions and billions of bits of information and experience we pick up through our bodies, hearts, senses and brains. It is complex and dynamic. It cannot be taken apart into individual components and reassembled like a car. Rather, it is complex – like a rainforest that follows its own logic to create a thriving ecosystem. It brews, moulds and sculpts stuff that we are unconscious of but may later be able to put into words. The *sea within* cannot be put into boxes, because then it ceases to flow. It is now time to dive into what we really mean by 'a state of flow' and how 'flow' is directly connected to the natural circulation of our InnSæi and enhances its powers.

A flow state is 'the deepest form of attention human beings can offer,' writes Johann Hari, the author of *Stolen Focus* (2022). When we are fully immersed in a feeling of energised focus, we become one with what we are doing, and we talk about being 'in the zone'. A flow state is an optimal state of consciousness, in which we feel and perform at our best. Alfred Gislason, one of the most successful handball club coaches in Germany and the coach of the national team, knows this feeling well. When I interviewed him, he said, 'Just before a game is thrown on it sometimes happens that I literally fall into the game. Everything else around me disappears. I only live in the game.'

He does not notice people in the audience, even if they make a point of speaking to him directly. 'Once an acquaintance complained to a mutual friend that he had approached me on the sideline of the field during a game in Berlin to say hi. I had acted as if I didn't know him. When my friend mentioned this to me I had no recollection of having seen him.' Alfred's immersion in the game is so complete that even his neurons begin to fire and his body moves as if he himself were playing the game.

An Austrian sports coach specialising in neurons once

commented to Alfred that his behaviour on the sideline during a handball game is one of the most extreme example of mirror neurons in action he has ever seen. Mirror neurons basically mirror the actions and behaviour of others – your body feels as if the other person's actions are your own. When I first heard about mirror neurons, it made me smile because I remembered how I tend to pick up behaviour from friends or even from people I don't know. Think about how you yawn when you see others yawn – and smiling can also be contagious. There is more research to be done in this field, but it seems that learning, empathy and compassion may all depend on a system of mirror neurons. The same principle may also apply to the destructive, violent and aggressive mental processes we experience or consume. This is how powerful those tiny neurons are.

As a pioneer, Mark Pollock is exploring the frontiers of spinal cord injury recovery through aggressive physical therapy and robotic technology. In 2016 he was able to walk with the help of electrical pulses and robotic exoskeleton. The movement stimulated his heart rate up to an aerobic training zone, a rate he had not even come close to since being paralysed. Like Alfred Gislason, Mark Pollock is an incredibly inspiring leader who shares his lessons generously with people from all over the world. When I asked Mark how he would describe intuition, or InnSæi, he said the first thing that came to mind was a gut feeling. But the more he thought about it, he felt that didn't quite capture the essence of it; it was much rather the altered state of consciousness found in 'flow', which he has been training to get into on demand. 'As part of that research and practice I have learned that our neocortex shuts down so that we lose our sense of self, time dilates – speeds up or slows down – things become effortless, and perhaps most relevant to your question we start to perform physically and mentally in a way that we didn't quite know we were capable of.' While Mark is coming from a perspective of exploring our performance potential through a flow state, he has discovered how that heightens our intuition in the process. This means that harnessing flow state to reach our fullest potential is done by enhancing our intuition and putting 'the editor' in our minds aside. The critical voice that is constantly commenting on how and what we are doing and drawing assumptions about the ability to achieve or do what we aspire to. This is one of the most common stoppers to the creative flow of writers, artists or anyone who wants to speak from the heart or take a leap of faith. A flow state, Mark continues to explain, allows us to be hyper-connected with ourselves, other people and the world around us. This, says Mark, is possible in 'a flow state where we perform unconsciously or intuitively in ways that we can't when our sophisticated pre-frontal cortex of our brains is taking over and making us overly rational and logical.'

Mihaly Csikszentmihalyi is probably the best-known expert in the area of flow. He is renowned for his seminal book, *Flow: the Psychology of Optimal Experience*, in which he outlined his theory that people are happiest when they are in a state of flow and completely absorbed in a challenging but doable task. At these times, they are so involved in the activity that nothing else matters; they are 'in the zone' or 'in the groove'. Their pre-frontal cortex function has been reduced, which means they have put their judgemental, overly analytical and doubtful inner critic aside, in order to perform at their best.

Not only does flow raise our levels of happiness and well-being, it also increases our creativity and productivity. In Csikszentmihalyi's words, flow is 'a state in which people are so involved in an activity that nothing else seems to matter; the experience is so enjoyable that people will continue to do it even at great cost, for the sheer sake of doing it'. The sea within them is flowing and not boxed in. They are in sync with Bruce Lee's metaphor on water – when nothing within them stays rigid the world opens up to them. Happiness is not a rigid, unchanging state, Csikszentmihalyi has argued. On the contrary, the manifestation of happiness takes a committed effort.

*I believe there is deep meaning in the world
for us to discover, not invent. It's a matter of
changing our attitudes and disposition towards
the world. Rather like tending the garden,
the plants will come up in their own time.
99.5 per cent of things going on around us are
now commonly accepted as being unconscious.
It's not a bad thing. This is where all the really
rich stuff is going on. It's important to liberate
people's intuition.*

INTERVIEW WITH IAIN MCGILCHRIST,
AUTHOR AND PSYCHIATRIST

McGilchrist maintains we are stuck in logic and rational thinking, at the cost of being more present, intuitive and connected to the world we live in. The Master is the vast, unconscious, intuitive, holistically perceptive mind, and the Emissary is the servant that helps realise the Master's mind through its ability to organise, analyse, calculate and execute. Over time, the Emissary, our rational, logical mind, has misunderstood his place in the world and now thinks he is the Master. Consequently, Iain argues, this has fundamentally disconnected us from a broader and more open approach to the world. Broadly speaking, the right hemisphere of the brain is characterised as the Master in Iain's book, and the Emissary the left hemisphere.

The difference between the hemispheres lies not in *what* they do, but *how* they do it.

'For evolutionary reasons we have had to be able to attend to the world in two different ways. We need to be able to relate to the world at large, at the same time as manipulating it. We need both of these approaches to the world, the narrow-focused one and the broad, open, sustained vigilant one,' he explained in the film *InnSæi*. The narrow-focused one is not unimportant – on the contrary, it is very important to help us organise information and knowledge, calculate, plan and analyse to name a few. But the negative side is that it has taken over our ability to be in a state of flow or see the big picture, to be present in the moment, intuitive and creative, understand how everything is interconnected and part of a complex whole, according to Iain McGilchrist.

Arguably, most of us are trained to explore the world and navigate it using a siloed approach. This means that we divide knowledge into different disciplines, which often do not even cross-fertilise to create a holistic view of the world. Every ten seconds an academic paper is published – amounting to about three million papers a year. Each one takes a long time to research, peer-review and finalise. A lot of energy, hours and resources are put into these research papers, and it is not even certain that they will be read by more than a handful of people. For instance, more than

70,000 papers have been published on a single protein, called 'p53'; and there are more than 10,000 papers on algorithms for self-driving cars, say Johan Rockström and Owen Gaffney in their book *Breaking Boundaries: The Science of Our Planet* (2021).

'With so much information flying around in so many disparate journals, largely locked behind paywalls, research can seem confusing, fragmented, unstructured, and impossible to keep up with, even for the experts who live and thrive in that world,' Rockström and Gaffney write. In the book *The Human Quest* (2012), Johan Rockström and Mattias Klum maintain that we not only need to reconnect with Earth to ensure sustainability and necessary mind-shift, but also enhance our creativity, intuition and expanded consciousness. InnSæi is a catalyst for cross-pollination, where things that may at first seem unrelated start to create cosmos out of chaos and the world opens up anew. From within the *sea within*, we are better able to see how everything is part of a greater whole.

The wayfinders

As we isolate, deconstruct, even celebrate these specific intellectual and observational gifts, we run the risk of missing the entire point, for the genius of Polynesian navigation lies not in the particular but in the whole, the manner in which all of these points of information come together in the mind of the wayfinder.

WADE DAVIS, *THE WAYFINDERS* (2009)

Consciousness and the ocean both have a fundamental impact on our existence, energy and intelligence on the one hand, and the weather, air and the food supply on the other. And yet both the ocean and consciousness remain largely a mystery. Is this because they are too intangible and immaterial, impossible to measure in a linear, statistical way? Is it because our methods and tools to comprehend the world we live in today are limited to the Emissary's frame of mind? Has it always been this way?

Hundreds of years ago, the ancient Polynesian navigators were able to map almost the entire Pacific Ocean without any of the technology we now have available to us. Today, even with the benefit of modern technology, it is estimated that we are only familiar with between 5 and 20 per cent of the world's oceans.

Our brains are wired to the world around us and it matters whether we observe life remotely, in an abstract or disconnected way, or if we immerse ourselves in it and allow it to inform us from the inside out. In Dalian, China in 2011 I met my friend, the ocean explorer Enric

Sala, for the first time. He used to be an academic but now spends most of his time underwater, exploring the ocean first-hand.

Enric grew up close to the sea in Spain and admired the leading 20th-century ocean explorer, filmmaker and conservationist Jacques-Yves Cousteau. Inspired by Cousteau's work, Enric studied marine biology and became a university professor. Having spent a while in the ivory towers of academia, Enric felt remote from the object of his passion, the ocean. In his own words, he resigned from his position at the university after he saw himself writing an obituary about ocean life. He saw the ocean's health degrade, sometimes to the point of extinction, and he felt an urgent desire to restore its ecosystems and ability to thrive. To do that, he needed to immerse himself in the ocean as much as possible, to sense its logic and help restore its powers. Today, Enric leads the National Geographic's Pristine Seas project, which has to date helped to create 26 of the largest marine reserves on the planet, covering an area of more than 6.5 million square kilometres. As he explained when I interviewed him, his work has helped him to 'develop this intuition about what's wrong with the ocean today and how to bring it back'. Not only was he inspired by Cousteau, but also by the ancient Polynesian navigators.

*I love the example of the Polynesian navigators,
where these people in small canoes travelled for
hundreds of miles on unknown, uncharted oceans
without knowing where they were going. They had
an amazing amount of knowledge... They knew
the waves, the currents, the clouds, the winds, the
stars. They could read the state of the sea. They
could know if there was an island in the distance
because of the reflection on a cloud. So, they had
this intuition about whether there was land, where
they were going. The Polynesians had collected
that massive amount of knowledge over many
generations and it became part of their collective
unconscious. They were able to map almost the
entire Pacific Ocean, which is the biggest ocean
area on Earth, without any modern technology
or GPS. Instead, they had stick charts. They were
able to do that only because they spent so much
time experiencing the ocean first-hand.*

ENRIC SALA, FROM THE FILM INNSÆI – THE SEA WITHIN

The story of the Polynesian navigators started ten centuries
before the birth of Christ. Five centuries before Columbus,
the Polynesians had over the course of only 80 generations
settled on virtually every island group of the Pacific,
establishing a single sphere of cultural life encompassing

some 25 million square kilometres. Most of the islands are relatively small and when you are sailing in the Pacific you see nothing but the vastness of the ocean and the endless skies.

Imagine for a moment what these journeys entailed. The sailors travelled in small, open canoes, all built with tools made from what nature provided, such as coral, stone and human bone. 'Their sails were woven from pandanus, the planking sewn together with cordage spun from coconut fibre; cracks were sealed with breadfruit sap and resins,' as Wade Davis describes in *The Wayfinders* (2009). 'Exposed to the elements, the sun by day, the cold wind by night, with hunger and thirst as constant companions, these people crossed thousands of kilometres of ocean, discovering hundreds of new lands, some the size of small continents, others mere island atolls less than a kilometre in diameter with no landmarks higher than a coconut tree.'

The ancient Polynesian navigators could 'pull islands out of the sea,' writes Wade Davis, with their extraordinary connection to the ocean and the natural world. They understood the physics and metaphysics of waves, could name between 200 and 300 stars and understood the meaning of constellations for wayfinding.

In recent years this ancient knowledge has resurfaced with people like Nainoa Thompson, president of the Polynesian Voyaging Society. Members of the Society have been training the younger generations to navigate based on the old traditions, remembering their cultural roots and the ways of their ancestors.

When I met one of Nainoa's collaborators, Tua Pittman, while sailing in the Pacific Ocean, I asked him about this work and we talked about InnSæi in the ancient and modern world. Tua spoke in a matter-of-fact manner about how we choose what we pay attention to and upload into our consciousness. We can deliberately immerse ourselves in the world and nature and navigate based on how this informs our InnSæi, or we can be the object of external navigational forces, like marketing, social media and man-made data. It is up to us, says Tua Pittman.

When you and I woke up this morning, we woke up under the same moon and stars as the ancient Polynesian navigators. What kind of world could we live in today, if we could connect with it using all our senses, from the sea within?

The wayfinders had to process an endless flow of data, intuitions and insights derived from their observation and the dynamic rhythms and interactions of nature around them. They were highly aware and aligned with their InnSæi and inner compass as they navigated the largest ocean on Earth. As Wade Davis explains eloquently in his book, *The Wayfinders*, their genius lay in comprehending the big picture and how everything comes together to create a whole. The ancient Polynesian navigators showed as much brilliance, says Wade, as mankind did when we sent a man to the moon. How we navigate and attend to the world matters. It will unravel the world before us, define our place in it and shape the way we affect it.

Main keys to InnSæi:

* The ocean is the oldest metaphor for consciousness. The deeper we go, the calmer both are. Our knowledge of the ocean and consciousness is limited; both are there for us to discover.

* Meditation and mindful breathing can help us reach the depths of our InnSæi and clarity of mind.

* The more deeply we connect to the *sea within*, the better we can connect with others and the world around us.

* We communicate beyond words and through our presence.

* Very few of our mental processes are conscious – in fact only a tiny fraction. Practise moving your spotlight of attention around, lighting up the world around you. When you do this, you are activating your InnSæi.

* Notice and be present with the animate, living part of the world; absorb its beauty and feel how it lights you up.

* Be like water – activate the *sea within* and outward things will disclose themselves.

* If the *sea within* is put into boxes or becomes rigid, it ceases to flow. Protect its flow.

* Flow is the deepest form of attention human beings can experience. Practise being completely absorbed in a challenging but doable task; practise putting your self-conscious, analytical inner critic aside. A flow state makes us happier, more creative and productive.

* InnSæi helps us cross-fertilise, see the big picture, and put things in context.

* How we navigate the world informs our place in the world and defines what we find.

Chapter 4

To see within
selfawareness helps harness your InnSæi

While our attention is fundamental to our ability to see within and access our InnSæi, it is an incredibly scarce resource. This is partly because we can be consciously aware of only a fraction of all the data coming our way every moment of every day, but it is also because our limited attention is highly sought after by external market forces which constantly strive to optimise their access to it. This can be quite challenging to deal with – not least because most of the time we aren't fully aware that it is taking place.

How we pay attention, and what we pay attention to, shapes how we experience the world we live in, act and imagine possibilities. Attention is what the 1978 Nobel Laureate in economics, Herbert A. Simon, called 'the bottleneck of human thought'. He coined the term 'attention economy', referring to the fact that our attention is a limited resource which is in high demand by a trillion-dollar market.

Your headspace is a lucrative market

We had better understand what is happening and make up our minds about it [new technologies] before it makes up our minds for us.

YUVAL NOAH HARARI, *HOMO DEUS* (2015)

The attention economy has been growing fast and relies on access to our personal headspace. Market forces are fully aware of our inability to pay attention to more than a fragment of the information flow and entertainment coming our way. And the flow of information has been accelerating in recent decades. It was only in 1993 that the world wide web or the internet, as we know it, was born; and today social media has about 4.89 billion users worldwide (as of August 2023). Over three billion people use Facebook, which is more people than follow Christianity, the world's most popular religion. Over five billion individuals use the internet now, which is over 64 per cent of the global population, according to Statista.

We buy, sell, communicate, learn, do business, and keep in contact with friends and family through online channels and screens; we also use them to build our profiles and even our identities. Entertainment, random videos and images we see online can educate and lift our spirits or have the opposite effect. Somewhere in between are hours spent watching and scrolling through images and videos that may leave no impact whatsoever. After hours or days without any likes or hearts on our social media postings, we may even find ourselves posting again, just to get reactions, as if we are double-checking that we really exist. Many of us are addicted to our online presence, which feeds extremely well into the income-generating strategies of businesses that are competing for our attention. The more scrolling we do, the more income they get, no matter what the content. In the attention economy, every second counts. The longer a brand can hold a customer's attention, the better it is for their bottom line. More attention means more sales.

- **Think about two things you do without thinking about doing them every morning. Things you do on autopilot, like brushing your teeth, putting on socks or going to school or work.**

- Next time you wake up, pay careful attention to how you are doing these two things.
- Notice what you notice and write it in your journal.

The algorithms behind some of this technology even micro-target our feelings, such as fear and vulnerability, to the extent that they have helped sway democratic elections and sparked destructive behaviour and deteriorating health among teens, especially girls. A US study covering 2001–2018 shows a striking correlation between the increasingly poor mental health of young women and girls and the rise of social media, especially from 2012 and 2013. The rise is measured in increased incidences of self-poisoning, suicide, major depressive episodes and depressive symptoms.

A lot of the time, perhaps most of the time, we are not even aware of how social media algorithms lead us on, sometimes down a rabbit hole of destructive thoughts or polarisation. Instead of self-regulating our attention, we hand it over to those who direct it where they will. We become more easily persuaded and – depending on what others want us to do – we scroll more or buy more. Meanwhile, we are feeding our mental processes with stuff that shapes our outlook on life.

Fragmented attention

The world seems like a heap of fragments and it's hard to see how they cohere. The sort of understanding that used to enable us to see what things mean has been lost so that wisdom has been replaced by knowledge and knowledge has been replaced by information, pieces of data, chunks of data.

IAIN MCGILCHRIST, IN THE FILM *INNSÆI*

It's no wonder the world seems fragmented. There are various studies and speculations out there, that explore to what extent the human attention span is changing and shrinking with fast paced technological advancement and information overload. Time will tell how much this is to the detriment of our brain power and intellectual capacity in the long run, given our mental ability to adapt, and also development of methods and ways for us to comprehend information, for example with artificial intelligence. Adam Hayes, an analyst and writer on Wyzowl, refers to a study which shows that the average office worker checks their email inbox on average every two minutes and checks their phones more than 200 times a day. According to a *Forbes* article some people are exposed to up to 4,000 and 10,000 advertisements a day, and people around the world spent on average around six and a half hours online, according to *Digital 2023: Global Overview Report*. And globally we spent on average about two hours and 15 minutes a day on social media in 2022, according to Statista.

A SIMPLE TECHNIQUE TO HELP RETAIN YOUR ENERGY AND SHARPEN YOUR FOCUS

- Our ability to focus decreases when interrupted. So set an alarm every 20 or 30 minutes, in order to stay focused on one thing at a time. It could be longer or shorter. The main thing is to train yourself to be focused on one thing at a time, to train yourself to maintain sustained attention. This will make you more engaged and improve your focus.

- The task may be anything – cleaning your home, attending to your kids, friends or family, writing or responding to emails, writing a text for a report, website, a letter to a friend, a book or an essay. Whatever it is, take five minutes or longer before you start again and use those minutes to scroll on your smartphone if you feel you need to do it, to eat or drink, call a friend or whatever you feel you need to do.

- **Decide to spend a maximum of seven minutes on social media a day.**

Our brains and senses seriously struggle with all this information. The 'Attention Deficit Crisis' podcast episode on the *Chasing Consciousness* website has some great insights from the host and his guest Johann Hari, author of *Stolen Focus*. Citing Professor Earl Miller, a neuroscientist at the Massachusetts Institute of Technology (MIT), Johann explains that while the average US teenager now believes they can follow six or seven forms of media at the same time, the reality is that we can consciously only think about one or two things at a time. When we are juggling many things at once, we do everything less competently, we make more mistakes, and we are less creative.

Another study found that the intelligence of people who are chronically interrupted by emails or phone calls is lowered by twice the rate it is lowered when we get stoned, Johann explains. Professor Earl Miller told Johann, that as a result we now live 'in a perfect storm of cognitive degradation'.

Beyond the overload of information, distraction and various demands that are thinning and fragmenting our attention, studies also show that chemical pollution can cause various neurodevelopmental disorders or IQ loss. This is why lead has been banned from paint and gasoline, and research continues to develop around environmental pollution and how it affects our well-being. Professor Barbara Demeneix, the author of *Losing Our Minds* (2014), who has studied some key factors that can disrupt attention and is an expert on the effects of chemical pollution, told Johann bluntly: "There is no way we can have a normal brain today." (see Notes)

It is worth bearing in mind that not all the studies mapping our ability to notice and process information come from researchers interested in enhancing or safeguarding human intelligence. Many others are carried out by marketing professionals, who are interested in finding ways to catch as much as possible of our attention to prolong the hours we spend online and raise their own revenue.

Can you see me? Can you see yourself?

When we spend face-to-face time, our presence and attention are among the greatest gifts we can give one another; and they help strengthen our relationships. In contrast, technology can drive us apart and isolate us in front of our screens. We see the consequences of this, and they have been documented in a growing number of studies that show that the less eye contact children have with their parents, the less they are able to establish relationships with others. Empathy has been declining and a 2018 study showed that attention deficit disorders in children and adolescents have been on the rise in the US in the last three decades. Unless we consciously guard our attention, we become immersed in content that respects no boundaries when it comes to things like false news, violence, polarisation or the age of the viewer.

There's a lot of pressure on us in today's world for reasons we do not fully comprehend. Many studies show how loneliness and isolation are making us unwell, both mentally and physically; we are also under a lot of pressure that comes both from around us and from within us. According to the World Health Organisation, depression is a leading cause of disability and illness in the world, and globally people are increasingly burning their candles at both ends. Regional, national and workplace studies show that the majority of people surveyed have experienced burnout at their current jobs and increasing levels of stress. Sometimes it is the younger generation (the 18- to 24-year-old) who feel the greatest impact.

Burnout is a state of emotional, physical and mental exhaustion caused by excessive and prolonged stress. It occurs when you feel overwhelmed, emotionally drained, unappreciated and unable to meet constant demands. Burnout is a gradual process; it doesn't happen overnight and the more you pay attention to your body and mental state, the more clearly you can see the signs and symptoms in good time and will be able to actively take care of yourself. Knowing yourself and regularly checking in with your InnSæi and body battery is key to understanding how you can take responsibility for your health.

Feeling aligned to your InnSæi and your personal values at work also matters. A recent survey on 'conscious quitting' confirms this. It was conducted among 4000 workers in the US and the UK and shows that most of them want to work for a company that is having a positive impact on the world. The survey also shows that one-third of these employees have resigned from their jobs because their values do not align with those of the company they work for.

Experiencing too much stress and anxiety, for too long, makes our brains turn to fight-or-flight mode, causing our mindset to shrink to 'tunnel vision'. This inhibits our creativity and decreases our sense of compassion and our ability to listen intently and focus deeply.

BREATHING EXERCISE

- When our brains are in fight-or-flight mode, we are stressed and short-breathed, we develop tunnel vision, lose sight of the context of things, are less (or not at all) creative and have less compassion.
- Breathing tunes our antenna, by regulating our neurosystem, which encourages the brain to be more open, receptive, compassionate and creative. Remind yourself to take a few deep breaths from morning to evening, at home, in meetings or while going from one place to another.
- Breathe in through your nose, and out through your mouth. Begin by counting to from 1 to 3 on the inbreath.
- The outbreath should be twice as long. You can prolong the outbreath by narrowing the space for air to go out of your mouth.
- Take a moment to feel how this calms you down.
- When you feel as if you are losing focus or control in a situation, try saying your name in your mind, like this: 'Hi (your name) ☺' This reminds your mind to stay inside your body and reminds you to stay connected to your soul in the moment.

Attending to the world in two different ways

As we saw in Chapter 3, the ancient Polynesian navigators were able to map almost the entire Pacific Ocean by immersing themselves in the ocean and the natural environment, an achievement unmatched to this day. There is a lot to be said about how we choose to wayfind in today's world, but to regain ownership of our own attention and focus let's recall the two fundamental ways in which we attend to the world, which we touched on earlier.

In order to shift our mindset and see *from the inside out*, we need to give our InnSæi a seat at the steering wheel. We know the whole body is our source of intelligence and it picks up data through our cells, senses and electromagnetic fields. We also know the brain is the central hub for processing, interpreting and directing our bodily functions, movement, mental states and actions.

Both hemispheres do similar things and they often substitute the other's function if need be, but as we have explored in Iain McGilchrist's work, evidence suggests they attend to the world differently. As we saw earlier, the difference lies not in *what* they do, but *how* they do it. The argument is that our over-emphasis on the left brain take on the world, the rational, analytical, logical and abstract lens, has been to the detriment of our ability to activate the full capacity of InnSæi and the right hemisphere.

The right hemisphere is in many ways home to our InnSæi since it sees the world as coherent, constantly moving, animate, flowing and complex and where nothing is completely separate from anything else. This 'kind of attention' is building a relationship between you and that world, between the things that are in that world. So you see a web of connections that are constantly changing,' Iain explained. The right hemisphere understands the implicit in the things not verbalised, it reads between the lines and recognises patterns. 'The left hemisphere,' however, 'pays this highy focused, narrowly targeted attention to something it wants to get. For the left hemisphere there are just fragments, little bits of things, and they are isolated and they don't connect with anything else. So one of the hemispheres is seeing the big picture and keeping with the continuity of our experience, while the other one is selecting a target within it and going for it. Now if you use that kind of attention to the world all you see is targets, things to grab, things to get.' The manner in which the left hemisphere attends to the world is abstract, static, inanimate, and according to Iain McGilchrist, it is so convinced of its own worth, that it has begun to take over. The right hemisphere sees the world as 'something living and ultimately never fully knowable, whereas the left hemisphere thinks it knows everything – *because it knows so very little.*'

We have become so caught up in the narrow, shallow and abstract thought processes of the left brain hemisphere, he argues, that we are losing the ability to sense the whole, inexhaustibly, truly wondrous, creative, living universe. Even our ability to feel a deep sense of awe has measurably decreased in the last decade, a theme we will explore in more depth in the next chapter. This imbalance translates into us perceiving the world as fragmented and siloed, we can't see InnSæi for what it is – nor embody its logic. We become discouraged from trusting and following it, as it is considered to be misleading and unscientific.

To summarise, Western culture has long relied on tangible metrics, and our ability to compartmentalise knowledge. This has led to our view of the world becoming fragmented. Meanwhile, the whole animate, interconnected world is right there in front of us. We can see how this translates into conventional healthcare services, where there is often a lack of understanding of mind-body connections; the body is seen as a collection of organs and parts, instead of an interconnected, complex whole. Similarly, our education systems compartmentalise our learning into disciplines and measure our competencies with easily comparable methods that fit analysis, statistics and reason, but not divergent thinking, creativity, InnSæi and imagination. The list goes on.

There will be more on the two different ways of attending to the world in the next chapter but, for now, let's continue with attention. Our purpose is to see within in order to witness and harness the magnificent sea within us.

Reaching the core of our being

It takes discipline and conscious intention to hear our inner voice and see within. Philosopher Matthew Crawford, author of *The World Beyond Your Head* (2015), talks about the value of silence in helping us control and own our attention. As clean air makes it possible to breathe, silence enables us to connect within and better access the sensory world. Silence in this context is not just about the noise and distractions in our environment; it also has to do with our ability to silence inner chatter, correct mistaken biases and beliefs, and peel off various filters in our heads, until we can reach the core of our being and harness our inner compass. It is only when we reach the core of our being that we can express ourselves authentically.

We will explore five different ways, or rituals if you like, that help us see within. They are:

1. Daily journaling
2. Mind the inflow to improve the outflow

3. Practise attention journaling
4. Take time for yourself
5. Broaden your horizon through grounding

1. Daily journaling

Journaling is powerful way to clean the space in your head and witness yourselves unfold. Journaling is simply about writing down your thoughts, feelings and ideas to acknowledge them and to understand them more clearly. It is often said that when we handwrite things, we are more likely to remember and register them. It is a great way to support your soul's flow and generate creativity. Nothing is set in stone or remains stagnant; even going to a meeting is an act of creativity; there is no script. Everything is subject to change and we are constantly co-creating everything, from conversations to actions, as we go through the day and our lives. No matter what your sphere of work, whether you are a student, an artist or lawyer, teacher or entrepreneur, journaling will sharpen your pencil and voice in the world. If you feel anxious, stressed or overwhelmed, journaling is a great way to express yourself and help release difficult emotions. Journaling is also a great way to capture creative ideas, solutions, or things you suddenly remember, whether it's day or night. This is why I highly recommend you carry a journal with you wherever you go, and have one at your bedside table if you wake up in the middle of the night wanting to write down an idea or something from a dream. Dreams can convey to us something important about our state of mind, feeling for things, or give us great ideas or funny stories. You can also write on your phone or save voice messages, although I wouldn't recommend screen time right before sleep or during the night.

The time to journal is always right, no matter if it's only a few minutes or longer, morning, midday or evening. But as with everything else, the more we practise, the more effective journaling becomes. Our brains are very open and trainable in the mornings when our brains wake up from a theta state, so journaling in the morning can be a powerful habit. But it can be very effective to do in the evening too, to clear our minds by putting thoughts onto the paper and leave it there for the night. As you will read in the last chapter of this book, evening journaling or journaling at the end of the day can also be a great habit to acknowledge what you have learned and done over the day, writing things down that you are grateful for, or that have inspired you in some ways. If you want to dive into the mastery of journaling to enhance your creativity, I highly recommend Julia Cameron's best-selling and classic book, *The Artist's Way* (2002).

Once we begin to journal we often start to be more aware of voices in our heads. From the world of writing, we often talk about the editor or censor, the perfectionist or overly-analytical, or logical voice that does not like what we are writing or thinking. When we journal, it's important to consciously decide that this voice needs to leave our headspace. It sometimes helps to be playful about it, and ask that voice politely to leave, it is not needed at this point. Other voices will pop up, too, and it is important to recognise them in order to find your own. We all have stories in our heads, based on old beliefs and assumptions. Some of these beliefs and assumptions may come from loved ones or may even be something we think loved ones would say, but we don't really know. When the brain predicts outcomes from old mental models, it reinforces a loop. Our mission is to make a hole in our mental model, step out of our habitual thinking and behaviour, and create space for new visions and ideas. Journaling can be an important step to open up to Iain's right brain hemisphere and Julia Cameron's artist brain.

Journal every day for at least two weeks; aim for 12 weeks if you can. Allow the thoughts and words to flow from your mind, without judgement or editing. Every minute matters, just start doing it. And if you miss a day, continue the day after. Let it all out, no one will see your journal, it is just for you.

Notice your fears, your core negative beliefs and the voices in your head, saying things like 'I will disappoint my parents or spouse, I am not good at this, someone has probably done this before, I will never have enough money, I am not educated for this,' and so on.

Practise open-mindedness. Don't judge the thoughts that swirl around in your head – neither the negative, destructive ones nor the big, bold ones. If you can't be sincere with yourself, who can you be sincere with?

Embrace your jealous voice. It's a great indicator of what you know you can and want to be doing. You may think: 'I could do that...' when you hear what someone else has done; your stomach may knot up or you may feel irritated. When you start to do more of the things you would truly like to do but have been hesitant or afraid to try out, you become less jealous. You switch from the slightly bitter 'I could do that...' to a warmer and generous 'Well done, that person! I know only too well that doing something like this takes a lot of work and courage.'

We can only allow ourselves to be vulnerable, and express our creative voice, when we feel safe with ourselves. And we can only feel safe if we truly accept who we are, warts and all. If friends, a spouse, relatives or a colleague happen to make a negative remark about you (such as 'this isn't like you' or 'what makes you think you can do this') as they start to see signs of your progress, rest assured that these remarks have nothing to do with you, they are about the person remarking. Your courage, actions or views may challenge their sense of place and their boundaries regarding what they do and don't allow themselves to do. Also, remember that your loved ones are just as likely to celebrate the changes in you and make positive remarks about what they see. When they do, remember to say 'thank you' and own your progress.

Witness yourself unfold as you continue journaling. It will help you decide what is worth sticking to and what is not, what thoughts help you and which do not. If there are people in your close circle of family, colleagues or friends who bring out negative energy in you, you might need to distance yourself from them a while, and you can find a way to do that with kindness. This may be hard, but you need to take responsibility for your own energy, boundaries and time. This takes constant practice.

Writing down your thoughts as they flow onto the page will help you get to know yourself better and understand how your mood can affect your outlook on life in positive and negative ways, which people give you support or inspiration and which do not. Journaling will unveil recurring fears, dreams and ideas for you to notice, throw away or keep. The more you get to know yourself, the more aligned you become. And the more aligned you become with your true inner voice, the more you trust your experiences and the more present you become. And the more present you become, the more you can mindfully take responsibility for your own mindset, actions and reactions.

Remember to be kind to yourself, because inside our souls and truest selves lie our greatest strengths and vulnerabilities. These two seemingly opposite poles are in fact mutually reaffirming. Someone once said to me that in our deepest emotions we are always vulnerable as children and therefore we, the adults, need to protect, love and honour the child in us. This advice came at a time when I was more inclined to self-sabotage and tackling vulnerability with toughness. Adopting this approach was transformative. It takes courage to be yourself, so make sure you give yourself the loving support you would give yourself as a child. The more you learn to honour and love yourself, the less other people can erode the ground you stand on. You feel more secure and grounded.

2. Mind the inflow to improve the outflow

This ritual helps us mindfully renew the reservoirs of our mind and spirit by filtering what comes in, such as news media, social media and toxic communications.

Some of us believe that missing out on a day's news is one of the seven deadly sins or at least something that might embarrass us in conversations with other people, because we won't be on top of things. I know this personally, having worked as a journalist and written about global development and politics. It was part of my identity to be well informed about current events. I therefore resisted the idea of cutting out all news coverage; but I then reaped the benefits of trying this out, which is why I am recommending it to you. I created more space in my head and body, felt calmer, and found that my horizons expanded, and I began to notice things I hadn't noticed before. This also applies to social media scrolling, take a pause and feel what it gives you instead.

After the recession in 2008, I created and directed a university diploma programme called Prisma ('Prism' in English). It was a two-month cross-disciplinary course, designed to train students in creative and critical thinking and sharpen their InnSæi in times of uncertainty. The students were aged from 19 to 67 years old, with matriculation exams to PhDs and had varied work experience. Most of them had lost their jobs in what we called 'the bank collapse' in Iceland and felt deeply insecure about things like their status in society, how to pay their bills and what the future held. We kept the students busy with inspiring talks and lessons given by some of Iceland's finest entrepreneurs, artists, academics and business leaders. We even had the former president of Iceland share with us her views on what it means to be a citizen of the world.

Throughout the course, we made sure the students kept their consumption of news to a minimum, because the news media tended to bring a negative energy, a politically charged and often hostile narrative, and a monolithic flow of information that narrowed the scope of thinking, as opposed to opening up their horizons to possibilities and multiple futures. In the case of Prisma, we helped fill the students' minds with new ideas and fresh sensory data, and simultaneously made sure they constantly checked in on themselves with exercises and methods, some of which are presented in this chapter.

Mindfully filtering and choosing the inflow of stimuli and information enables us to align with InnSæi, release blockages and renew our energy. We feel more interested, and in return become more interesting to others.

3. Practise attention journaling

Iain McGilchrist has said that the way we pay attention to the world is a moral act. This is because the kind of attention we pay both changes the world we experience – the only world we can know – and changes ourselves. It is not a passive act but a relational encounter. He recommends practices that cultivate an active, open receptivity to the world. When we practise attention journaling, we are allowing the world to come into being before us, rather than 'driving it away with our preconceptions, self-righteous anger and ready judgement,' as Iain put it in our conversation for this book. I agree with him. With our attention we open up a world that is either alive or dead, a world where everything is either interconnected and animate, or inanimate and siloed. How we attend to the world changes us and the energy we emit from within.

The most powerful creative tool I know is 'pay attention to what you pay attention to, and document it'. My friend, the late artist and writer, Thorvaldur Thorsteinsson, gave it to me at the dawn of this century. It's a gift that keeps giving and creating ripple effects from within for everyone who practises it. Paying attention to what we pay attention to is a powerful way to witness ourselves and see within. Like journaling, documenting how we pay attention is transformative. It allows the world to come to us and enables us to witness it show up inside ourselves.

Attention journaling is about capturing what our attention brings us but we don't notice most of the time. We allow the world to come to us and observe ourselves from a distance. We become more open to the unexpected, the stuff that lies on the periphery of our focused mind and is difficult to put into words.

START ATTENTION JOURNALING

- Carry a journal with you for three weeks to begin with. Jot in it the things you pay attention to. You can use the same journal as you use for the daily journaling.

- Don't overthink it. Simply document what you notice during the day or in your dreams at night.
- Don't judge what your attention picks up. It is not yours to judge. Simply witness it.
- Attention journaling is not like a regular diary, where you write down what you had for breakfast or describe the weather each morning. You only write what your attention catches, and it may be individual words, such as 'bad smell', 'she wears her trouser to hide her body', 'I lost my breath over the beauty', 'flags outside shop in crayon colours', 'wired energy between two people at the till', 'warm smile and his reaction', 'her energy was (fill in)'. Pay attention to how you attend to people's presence, voice, energy or physical expressions; see it as a reflection on you, not them.
- InnSæi is embodied. Notice how you pay attention with your whole body and all your senses and jot down what you notice.

Creativity thrives on going into the unknown. If we know exactly where or how we are going, we are not being creative about the journey. In many ways, creativity is about seeing the world with fresh eyes, opening up our InnSæi, making the familiar strange, and the strange familiar. We wake up sleeping systems, the mundane becomes interesting, even magical and we start to care for it more.

CHOOSE TEN WORDS OR PHRASES

- At the end of each week of writing in your attention journal, flip through the pages and choose ten words randomly, and underline or highlight them.
- Now write out those notes or words in a vertical line on a fresh sheet of paper.
- Give yourself time to read this list, without judgement, and think: What do these words tell me? What is behind them?
- Each word and sense is there because you attended to it. Allow patterns, shapes, narrative or a feeling to emerge. Trust the process, let go of control, let context come to you.
- This is raw material for sense-making or artistic writing or ideas to emerge.

GET TO KNOW YOURSELF BETTER

For self-regulation and to get to know yourself better, read through your attention journal and mark the following in different colours. This will enable you to map your inner landscape over a period of one or three weeks, or longer if you wish.

Look out for:
- Toxic relationships
- Generous relationsips
- Recurring thoughts or ideas
- Your own prejudices
- Your fears and limitations
- What you notice in other people you pay attention to
- Your jealous moments
- And patterns emerging or recurring themes?

Recurring ideas, voices or patterns can be a source for new ideas, mindset or decisions.

4. Take time for yourself

As much as your colleagues want to encourage you to take personal time off or your loved ones love you, they might at some point ask if you can use this time to do something for the company, practical around the house, for the family, or start comparing their use of their time with yours. Remember, people usually see you through the lens of themselves. So when you are taking time for yourself, just say you are at a meeting, visiting a friend or at work.

Our days are so packed, we need discipline to create space for seeing within. At these dates, make sure you do something that nourishes your soul, body and mind. Something that creates headspace or silence, the condition of not being addressed. Do stuff that inspires you when you need inspiration or something that calms your nervous system when it feels wired. Do something open-ended, like walking in a forest or a park, because trees and the colour green calm our nerves. Sense the elements around you. Smell the pine trees, feel the wind on your skin, your body, in your hair. Hear the birds sing. If you are near the seashore, hear the soothing sound of the waves coming in and out, or stick your toes into the sand on the beach or the soil or wherever you find yourself.

Relatively broad horizons and landscapes open up our minds, oxygen calms us and fresh winds stir our souls and activate our energy. Go out and take some photos of what you see. You'll be surprised at what you come up with. Go to cafés and create stories in your head about the strangers you see there. Or stay inside, rest, take a bath or do a puzzle.

If you want to go outside but can't, try closing your eyes and imagining you are out in nature. You may want to try some of the practical exercises that appear throughout this book. Notice how taking time for yourself connects you to yourself.

5. Broaden your horizon through grounding

Grounding is a powerful way to align ourselves with InnSæi, to calm our systems and broaden our horizons. Let's imagine for a moment that we are individual trees that are part of a complex interconnected web.

Trees are magnificent beings that rise individually from the ground up, but below the surface of the earth they are part of a complex root system. Trees communicate, cross-fertilise and organise through their root system, which is usually below the surface of the earth and therefore out of sight. In some ways, they resemble our unconscious and the things in life that aren't visible, similar to our brainwaves and energy fields that cross-fertilise and have intangible ripple effects on others.

Trees in the rainforests play a critical role in stabilising Earth's weather systems by calling forth rain and turning carbon dioxide into oxygen. Around 70 per cent of the carbon they photosynthesise they take below ground, where their roots store it and trade the carbon for nutrients.

Fungi also play a really important part in stabilising carbon in the soil. Life on Earth is mostly made up of the same stuff as the stars in the skies. This includes the mycelium, the mother of us all, who climbed out of the sea about 4.5 billion years ago to create fertile soil and set the stage for all life on Earth. As the documentary film *Fantastic Fungi* (2019) explains, mycelia are networks of root-like fungal threads which branched into fungi and animals about 650 million years ago.

Mycelia can have literally trillions of end branches and they share a similar network design to the internet. Mycelia have more networks than our brains have neural pathways and they work in much the same way, by means of electrolytes and electrical pulses.

They are the most common species on Earth – they are literally everywhere. Trees use mycelia as pathways to communicate, connect and feed one another. Mycelia enable trees to feed and exchange nutrients; and when a tree is showing weakness, a mother tree will use its mycelia to send extra nutrients and support, like the love and support humans give each other every hour of every day somewhere in the world. Living creatures, like fungi and mycelia, are intelligent. They respond to the environment, solve problems, seek out food and defend themselves.

The family tree of humanity also turns out to be an incredible web of life that connects us more than we previously thought. As Wade Davis puts it in his book *The Wayfinders* (2009), 'Each one of us is a chapter in the greatest story ever written, a narrative of exploration and discovery remembered not only in myth but encoded in our blood'. While we can map family trees and the way humans have dispersed around the world through the centuries, we are also held in an invisible web of connections that we share not only through our bodies when we are in each other's presence, but also through generations, stored in memories of felt moments, lost and found hopes and other life experiences that have enabled our species to survive.

Our responses to social stimuli can cause changes in hundreds, sometimes thousands, of genes and have ripple effects both within and beyond our brains and bodies as books like Thomas Verny's *The Embodied Mind* (2021) illustrate. Verny points out that most geneticists and neuroscientists would not have believed all this even 20 years ago. This is how fast our knowledge is changing and expanding.

No matter how distantly related we seem, our roots on Earth can all be traced back to the same set of individuals; and all the people who co-exist with us now carry the genes of our common ancestors, says Susanna Manrubia, a theoretical evolutionary biologist at the Spanish National Center for Biotechnology.

On a recent visit to the Neanderthal Museum in Germany, I discovered that this is the first time in history that we, homo sapiens, find ourselves as the only human species on Earth and this is an evolutionary exception.

Instead of being seen as a family 'tree', our evolution is today thought of as a wide river, which can branch and form new streams that can later flow together once more. Human evolution is a creative process and the result of adaptation and chance. Our shared history is written in our bones, and as the anthropologist Wade Davis wrote so eloquently in *The Wayfinders*:

> *We are all literally brothers and sisters.*
> *Humanity's greatest legacy, the intellectual and*
> *spiritual web of life that envelops the planet, is*
> *the sum total of all our dreams, thoughts and*
> *intuitions, myths and beliefs, ideas and inspirations*
> *brought into being by the human imagination*
> *since the dawn of consciousness.*

What would the human legacy and the world look like if we were all consciously and deeply connected to and through our InnSæi like the web of mycelium throughout the millennia? How would we honour ourselves or interact with other beings and planet Earth differently?

GROUNDING EXERCISE

- Stand with both feet on the ground. Put your hands together at chest height, close your eyes and honour yourself and the ground you stand on.
- Extend your hands upwards to reach the sky. Imagine you are a tree, with branches, leaves and crown, rising gracefully from the Earth.
- Feel the soles of your feet and imagine they are sprouting roots deep into the centre of Mother Earth. Visualise your roots below the surface of the Earth, how they mix in with everyone else's roots and are a part of an interconnected, intelligent and mutually supportive human root system.
- See the centre of the Earth as a powerful ball of energy, fire and light. Visualise your roots connecting to this centre, and feel them tapping into it to fill themselves with its energy and nutrition.
- Witness your roots transporting this energy and nutrition all the way up again, from the centre of the Earth into the soles of your feet and from there into your whole body. You are standing strong, you can weather the storms of life because the Earth is holding you.

To summarise, InnSæi releases the power of goodness in communities that rely upon cooperation, flexibility and mutual support, much like the world of plants, especially roots, trees, mycelia and fungi. Evolution partly depends on mutual benefit and generosity. Within ecosystems there are plants, insects and living beings that support each other in different ways and they give and take while doing that. Fungis helps dead trees become soil again, trees in the rainforest will give way for higher trees to access the sun. When we see inside ourselves and feel this in our bones, we begin to understand, embody and care about it. We are shifting the centre of gravity inside us and balancing the world within us with the world around us. This enables us to become aligned with the interconnectedness of being. We are part of the same ecosystem and it is not clear where you end and I begin. When we experience the world as fragmented, it is because we have lost our innate sense of interconnectedness. We no longer feel we are an integral part of the world we live in. We are a fragment in a pile of fragments; and we lose our sense of belonging, purpose and kinship with other living beings.

Main keys to InnSæi:

* Your attention is a scarce resource and much sought after in today's economy.

* Attention is the key to seeing within and accessing our InnSæi.

* How we pay attention shapes how we act and imagine possibilities.

* It takes discipline and intention to be able to see within.

* Sustained attention deepens our InnSæi; shortened attention detracts from human intelligence.

* For evolutionary reasons, we attend to the world in two different ways. We can see the world at large, the context of things and how they interconnect, and at the same time we categorise information and manipulate it in order to survive and make plans.

* Make the five rituals to *see within* a part of your daily life. They are:

  ★ Journal regularly, in a stream of consciousness and without judgement; this will help you clear your way to your InnSæi.

* Take a break from news media, toxic relationships, social information and distracting information for a while. You need to empty your well in order to fill it. This will help you release blockages and renew your energy. Filter the inflow to improve your outflow.

* Pay attention to what you pay attention to and document it in your journal. This will light up your senses and enable you to align with your InnSæi, enhance your creativity and self-knowledge.

* Take time for yourself at least once a week.

* Broaden your horizons through grounding; witness yourself unfold from within and sense the interconnectedness of life.

Chapter 5

To See From the Inside Out

navigate with your InnSæi

The navigator must process an endless flow of data,
intuitions and insights derived from observation and
the dynamic rhythms and interactions of wind, waves,
clouds, stars, sun, moon, the flight of birds, a bed of
kelp, the glow of phosphorescence on a shallow reef
– in short, the constantly changing world of weather
and the sea...

WADE DAVIS, FROM *THE WAYFINDERS* (2009)

Two rhythms and a strong inner compass

The human spirit has its own circulation system to renew,
recreate and evolve. We know that InnSæi is embodied
and has its own rhythmic ebbs and flows; and the better we
harness those, the more creative, intelligent and grounded

we can become. Imagine we function in the interplay of two different rhythms which we seek to balance. One rhythm encompasses creativity, sensing, symbols and feelings. This is the one that takes deep breaths, receives and reflects. It enables us to feel present and to pay attention to what we pay attention to; it knows when to let go of control and trust the process. It is the subjective, experienced and sensed. It opens us up to the animate world and enables us to be inspired by it. In this rhythm, we are artists and explorers at heart.

The other rhythm is that of rational, deliberate, inanimate and analytical thinking. We rely on it to calculate, build houses, organise, create tools and plan for the storm. It enables us to quantify and measure. On its own, it has nothing new to say; it builds on what we already know and can measure. It can easily be mechanical, fragmented and act out of context with the rest of the world. This rhythm is a means to an end, not an end in itself. In short, it helps us get stuff done but it has little room for uncertainty, imagination, innovation or change.

For many of us, it takes a lot of self-discipline to let go of control, to be mindful and in the moment. For others it is the other way around – and it can take a lot of discipline to follow through on ideas and decisions, plan and decide. Everyone probably follows a combination of the two. The two rhythms and a strong inner compass is a metaphorical navigation tool for wayfinding in the complex universe inside and around us. The more we deepen and balance these two rhythms, the stronger our InnSæi and inner compass.

Our minds have been wired to give more credibility and emphasis to the rational, quantifiable, siloed and analytical thinking rhythm at the cost of the creative, animate, interconnected and intuitive one. We are led to believe that embodied experience and conscious perception are less reliable or important than the quantifiable realm of mathematics or science. As my daughter Rán pointed out when she was a 15-year-old student, 'If you are not good in physics or maths you are considered stupid. If you are not good in the arts it matters less, they say it's simply not your field.'

This matters, because the questions we ask, the answers we listen to and the way in which we use the results depend on our underlying beliefs and assumptions. This shows up in our siloed structures, from our schools and conventional healthcare systems to our economic models.

Reflecting on the research Dr George Land and Dr Beth Jarman did on creativity for NASA and how it showed that creativity reduces dramatically with age, Dr Land said: 'Look folks, if we're going to enter the future with hope, that's not going to work. We need to do something about it.' I agree with Dr Land and want to add that creativity is not just about our ability to innovate and rethink our business models, technology and systems. Creativity also connects us within and keeps our souls regenerated and inspired. It relies on InnSæi and has healing powers in itself.

I decided to resign from my permanent position at the United Nations – which had been my dream job – because I felt stuck in one rhythm, at the cost of the other. It wasn't the mission that bothered me: it was the structure of the work that dimmed my light, restrained my agency and drained my energy. I could see my own disconnection reflected in the system I was serving, a system that felt disconnected from the people and the planet it was meant to serve. The highly bureaucratic and hierarchical culture at the UN made me realise that we have created systems around systems, around systems, and lost sight of the real stuff, the heartbeat and warmth of real connection, the ground beneath our feet and how everything is linked.

A year and a half after my resignation I spent part of the summer on a small island in northern Iceland, where I started to write down my thoughts about the ideal approach to education, based on the experiences I have shared so far. Education, the way we prepare our kids for life and how we as adults keep learning throughout life, is fundamental to the path we choose and the questions we ask. My ideas developed into a university diploma programme when the bank collapse hit Iceland in October 2008. At this point, a huge number of people lost their jobs, savings and homes, and heads of universities and the Directorate of Labour were calling for new solutions to generate employment and rebuild our economy.

I decided to pitch my idea for an education module based on the two rhythms and a cross-disciplinary education and this quickly turned into Prisma (e. prism), a diploma programme at the Arts Academy of Iceland, the University of Bifrost and the Reykjavíkur Akademían. For each six- to eight-week module, around 40 experts, professors and cultural leaders shared their insights from dozens of disciplines and practices. There were case studies demonstrating innovation and entrepreneurship, and lectures in international relations, business, history, anthropology, cultural studies, philosophy, design, and the arts. Alongside this intensive and varied injection of knowledge and ways to interpret the world, the students were trained to sharpen their InnSæi and inner compass with methods and exercises, some of which I have shared in this book.

The students were aged between 19 and 67, with incredibly varied work experience, levels of education and background. Prisma opened their minds to new possibilities, enlarged their skillset and sharpened their direction in life. Some spoke about the healing effects of Prisma. I remember when one of my closest colleagues, one of four facilitators who led students through the Prisma methodology and assignments, came to me on the third week of the first module to share his personal experience of working in this environment. He said he felt less stressed, more loving and creative, and he could even feel the difference in his relationship with his wife. His words and experience echoed those of the French horse trainer Franck Mourier, described in Chapter 1, who shared with Iain McGilchrist that the more he honoured and harnessed his intuition, the more open and generous he became in spirit.

Prisma was about creating an enabling constellation, an environment that deepened and strengthened the two rhythms, and a strong inner compass. It was based on the belief that if we attend to and grow the soil in people and train them to activate their InnSæi in a critical and conscious way, meaningful and heartfelt ideas and directions will emerge from within them. Their inner compass will become strong enough for them to consciously carve their own way in a turbulent world.

To me, it was all about the vibe and the constellation of education and physical space we designed for students. If we could get that right, everything else would follow. My incredibly talented and diverse team and I made sure the curriculum and the facilitation of discussions and explorations took place in a secure environment, free from the politically charged atmosphere outside the doors.

Inside we emphasised keeping the interiors beautiful, we decorated with colourful fabrics and furniture, books and music. We delved into themes with a curious and critical mindset and trained ourselves to see the familiar with wonder and fresh eyes. Prisma was disruptive and unconventional enough to make people feel they were on the same boat, no matter what their previous position in life or work. In this case, the economic crisis in Iceland was truly the 'mother of invention' and enabler of new ideas, making it possible for Prisma to emerge.

Four steps in Prisma

We applied these four steps to all Prisma assignments and group discussions:

1. To see, feel and hear more.

2. To reverse – to make the strange familiar and the familiar strange.

3. To put into context – to create cosmos out of chaos, and find unexpected connections between seemingly unrelated parts.

4. To create on your own terms.

The value of intuition

Daniel L. Shapiro is the founder and director of the Harvard International Negotiation Program and a world-renowned expert on the psychology of conflict resolution. In his book, *Negotiating the Nonnegotiable* (2016), Daniel takes the reader into the heart of conflict, whether its families in crisis, warring political groups or disputing businesspeople. I was lucky enough to get to know Daniel while he was writing his book and, since then, we have discussed intuition in various contexts. While Daniel celebrates the fact that more people now recognise the key role intuition can play in the future of our planet, lasting cooperation and good decision-making, he still thinks 'we have a long way to go in fully recognising the power of intuition'.

Authentic leaders, visionaries, artists and changemakers navigate with a strong inner compass, expressed through their unique voice and impact in the world. They understand what a sense of alignment with InnSæi and balance between the two rhythms means and they honour that as their source of strength, resilience and direction. They are conscious of the importance of keeping their rhythms in balance through their InnSæi, whether they are pushing teams beyond what they think possible, catalysing collaborations to find a cure for paralysis in our lifetime, regenerating our ocean's ecosystems or helping people get grounded in their bodies.

For Alfred Gislason, the art of coaching is to help professional athletes reach their highest potential, both as individuals and as a team, beyond what they imagined possible. To this end, InnSæi is important for several reasons. When I interviewed him in 2022, he said, 'For me, InnSæi is what is called *Bauchgefühl* in German, a gut feeling or gut thought. The knowing that is simply there, shows up and tells you the right thing to do, even if you have nothing to support it yet. Perhaps this is an ability we have had from ages ago when our instincts were a defining factor in whether we lived or died. When sensitivity to the environment was a necessity for survival.'

Some people may be more open to listening to this inner voice and it seems that one can either enhance it or suppress it. Alfred continued:

> [Intuition] helps me release myself from my own plans and get a different perspective on things, to be open to the unexpected... If you are open to taking decisions based on your InnSæi and they turn out to be right more often than not, then you get more and more confident following it. But naturally the knowledge and experience we have plays an important role in how good our InnSæi

is. The people you work with also learn to trust in your hunches; at least if they more often than not have worked out for the team...

Emotional intelligence, the ability to 'see inside' the players and where they are coming from, is key to bringing out the best in a team, according to Alfred:

I need to understand what works best for each player, in what situation on the field they feel at their best, and when not. For this to work, it is important that I give myself time to establish a personal relationship with my players, to get to know them better and develop a better feeling and InnSæi about them, to be able to read into their behaviour from day to day. Players, like other people, vary when it comes to their preferences; what is unimportant for one person can be of fundamental importance for someone else. This kind of knowledge can help prevent misunderstandings and disputes within the team, which could if unaddressed have serious consequences for the team spirit.

For Alfred it's important to activate the team members to ensure there is strong ownership of the process. The players he has coached have come from different cultural backgrounds and speak different languages. 'They need to understand what we are doing and be willing to do what it takes to be successful.' During the second season when Alfred was coaching the Magdeburg handball team, he felt there wasn't a strong enough harmony in this understanding among the team players, so he decided to try a new strategy to strengthen their sense of ownership of the game plans.

He was used to doing most of the talking at tactical meetings with the team, where he explained different game plans for various circumstances. They all followed him with interest and focused attention, but he felt something was missing. So he decided to shift the roles in these meetings. After explaining each plan himself, he asked each player to describe to the others in the team what the game plan was, in their own words. He realised that each of them felt they understood perfectly what he was telling them 'but it turned out their understanding varied somewhat, which made a difference for us as a team.'

As a coach or a manager, you have to be interested in the people you are working with, their needs and unique positions within the group, he explains. You have to be willing to listen to everyone's point of view and respect what people want to discuss or ask about:

Relationships like that are built on mutual trust and sincere interest in the circumstances of everyone on the team. It is also based on my willingness to give of myself, to be generous with my experience and insights. When this works out well, it becomes easier and simpler to take decisions under pressure. Sometimes decisions I take might not seem rational in the moment, but because of this shared experience in the team, they make sense to us and they work...

I often spend an incredible amount of time analysing our opponents, I go through all the games of my own team thoroughly, especially those we lost or those that didn't work out as I would have wanted. It is work that often borders on being self-torture.

When he makes this comment about 'self-torture' he is referring to the detailed video analysis and editing of the games, which often continues late into the nights before the team plays their next game. Alfred does all the game analysis himself, which is in line with his belief that it is important to be immersed in the game. In the same way as his players need to be able to explain game plans in their own words and embody the tactics, he finds it crucial to go through the games himself manually and analyse and edit each one. This helps deepen his feeling for the game and the players in ways that would be impossible if he didn't do this work himself.

As a well-known coach and a former professional athlete, Alfred Gislason is used to working under pressure and often under public scrutiny. Although he enjoys the pressure that comes with high expectations of delivery and performance, he is also acutely aware of the importance of 'filling his tank' by finding a balance between the two rhythms. To this end, he seeks solitude in the countryside in Germany, where he gets grounded, cycles, tends bees, and grows roses, vegetables and fruit.

He sums all this up at the end of our conversation:

My experience has taught me that it is important to divert my attention away from what's pressuring me and the expectations about certain results, to things that slow down time, help me get grounded and let my mind flow. It helps me release myself from my own plans and get a different perspective on things, to be open to the unexpected.

I have always made sure to train regularly, and today I mostly cycle for 1.5–2.5 hours a few times a week. This is where I get most of my best ideas, when I am in fact not thinking about work.

And when he is at home he is always moving around, attending to his surroundings. 'I am building something, growing vegetables, trying to improve the soil through various experiments. I have bees, hens and I have been growing dozens of rare roses and fruit trees, some of which I have found on my cycling tours in the countryside. These have been both my hobbies and my ways to not burn out in my other world.'

The two rhythms often feel like two extremes for Alfred. When he has been away working a lot and comes home to relax and attend to his hobbies, he says, 'I feel time passes slower after a few days. I can feel how I get myself more grounded and connected to the things that matter most. It's a strange paradox because at the same time I consider myself an adrenalin junkie, because I also feel good when under pressure.'

A state of flow heightens our InnSæi

We first met Mark Pollock in Chapter 2. He is someone who has pushed the boundaries as an extreme athlete, seeks to find a cure for paralysis in our lifetime and helps other people perform at their best. Mark has developed a trainable way to optimise his alignment to InnSæi by switching between the two rhythms. His insights come from years of practice, research, coaching and writing, and his work with some of the world's finest physiologists, innovators and scientists. For the first few years after becoming paralysed, Mark offered himself as 'a guinea pig' for scientists to test new technologies and monitor his nervous system's reaction, on his mission to cure paralysis in our lifetime. Mark is also known for having developed an incredibly resilient and curious mindset which he helps people to adopt through his coaching and inspirational talks around the world. His knowledge base is therefore extensive, broad and embodied.

As we saw in Chapter 3, Mark uses a state of flow to access and activate his InnSæi. In the process of doing this, he started to perform physically and mentally in a way he hadn't realised he was capable of. 'When we're in flow,' he explains, 'we are able to perform unconsciously or intuitively in ways that we can't when our sophisticated neocortex or pre-frontal cortex is taking over, making us too logical.'

Intuition is telling us something we couldn't rationally state, by summarising it in a few points. Instead our intuition brings together information from our whole body – our senses, our inner being, our knowledge, our history – to find patterns to give us answers or clues. Shutting down parts of our brains and rooting ourselves inside our whole bodies is the key to attaining this higher level of performance. Mark continues, 'In my work to cure paralysis and through my sports background, I understand that our minds and bodies are connected, that our sensory and motor systems are connected in ways that we don't even fully understand yet. So, being connected inside and out is important and that's what flow states allow us to do.'

Mark goes on to explain the intelligence found in the whole body, taking the example of walking. Walking is something that most of us would consider a simple act but Mark Pollock understands too well that it is actually extremely complex:

The simple act of walking is not so simple. Hundreds of things are going on with the environment, your body and their dynamic interaction all at the same time. You can't follow it all consciously. The complex system required for walking cannot be done exclusively with the rational part of the brain. The big discovery about walking is that the brain is not controlling everything whenever we walk. In fact, we have many brains; at the bottom of our spine, the spinal cord is intelligent and has little to do with the brain. So, when I am trying to walk in my exoskeleton with spinal stimulation on, we are exploring if it would be better for me to consciously think about putting the right foot down, and at the same time lift my left leg and

engage my glutes, calves and so on? Arguably,
it is too complicated. Perhaps it would be better
to walk unconsciously? It is the lack of conscious
thought that enables the magic to happen and
that's what we access when we are in flow.

Accessing a flow state heightens our intuition and allows us to be 'hyper-connected with ourselves, other people and the world around us,' says Mark Pollock. 'If you are always switched on, executing and moving too quickly between people and places, you can only operate at a shallow level. This includes shallow reflection on yourself, connection with other people and the broader questions about the rest of the world.'

It requires discipline to find the space for
a lack of discipline
MARK POLLOCK

Today, Mark Pollock's work leans towards regular office work as opposed to the deserts and ice caps of his endurance racing, but he likes to organise it in the Olympic cycle of four years. He writes down annual key result areas, quarterly clear goals, weekly priorities and daily actions as he works towards his four-year plan. He uses what he calls a clarity stack with a 'why' statement at the top, narrowing from that broad 'why' to the specific daily actions required and back again. 'Everything I do is about inspiring people to build resilience and collaborate with others so that they achieve more than they thought possible. My 'why' statement helps me to rule projects in and out, based on the three pillars I have created for myself, which are resilience, collaboration and performance. Everything I do needs to fit those pillars,' he explains.

Clarity becomes one of the main triggers for being able to go into a flow state, because flow follows focus. Then we shut down the parts of the brain that make us stay in 'analysis mode' as opposed to 'doing mode'. A clearer framework creates more space for flow. Mark tries to be as specific as he can about weekly and daily actions. Roughly speaking, his days start with two hours of flow and writing. Then he exercises, goes back to a flow block without distractions for about one hour, has lunch, and uses the afternoons for meetings and calls that are more likely to be messy and more of a struggle, before he reviews the day, acknowledging what he has done.

Being specific about daily actions, he might aim to write themes for one of his talks, chapter headings for a book he is working on, or whatever it might be. 'The clarity stack also allows me a filter to say no to all the other projects that I could get excited about,' he explains. 'Basically, I'm trying to create filters, to release myself from the avalanche of opportunities and things happening in the world and reduce the cognitive load that I subject myself to so that I can perform better.' We can't do everything that's available to us. It's about navigating with our inner compass and being able to tell the difference between what is aligned with us and what isn't.

For many of us, it takes discipline to get ourselves into a state of flow or live a flow lifestyle. Besides being an excellent way to improve our performance and enhance our intelligence, flow also reduces stress, and regenerates and empowers our creativity. 'We actually need to create the space to do nothing and structure recovery in day-to-day life. It requires discipline to find the space for lack of discipline,' says Mark. And here's where his sports experience comes in handy:

As part of the flow cycle of struggle, release, flow and recovery, I know that dropping out of the flow state where you feel at your best can feel terrible. It is when all the addictive neurochemicals of flow disappear and you feel incapable of doing very much at all, never mind performing at a high level. This is when we must treat recovery like a high performance non-negotiable. It requires active recovery, like exercise, saunas, ice baths and sea swimming, or simply sleeping, relaxing and having a laugh.

Mark also goes out on his tandem handbike, to the gym and comedy nights. He may also go out for a brunch with friends, go to the pub, or listen to sports matches while relaxing and recovering:

Before I didn't realise the very nature of being a sportsperson automatically has rest and recovery and cycles built in within the season and post-season breaks. For many years, as a sportsperson I was living this struggle, release, optimal performance, recovery cycle. It wasn't just in a training context, but also after racing during the season and then when the season was over, with time for holidays. I didn't know about flow then, but I was living a flowy lifestyle where rest and recovery were built in.

CREATE YOUR OWN CLARITY STACK

- Define your 'why' statement and use it to decide how to prioritise your time and energy.
- Your 'why' statement gives you clarity and creates a framework for flow.
- The clearer the framework, the better your chances of getting into flow.
- Paths lead in all directions, but your 'why' will

- help you align to your InnSæi as your inner compass.
- Treat recovery as a high-performance non-negotiable. For the tough cookies and perfectionists out there: fun recoveries with lots of laughing are effective too!

Creativity is a state of mind

Before, Mark was not used to thinking of himself as a creative person, but flow has opened up his creativity and enabled him to come up with answers he didn't realise he had. 'We start to make creative connections in ways we simply can't when we're being overly rational and logical,' he says.

Mark came across a Red Bull research project from 2015, called 'Hacking Creativity', where they reviewed more than 30,000 scientific studies and conducted hundreds of interviews with experts. The study intrigued him as it found that creativity is the most important skill for success in our fast-paced world. 'Unfortunately, the other thing they discovered,' said Mark, 'was that it is extremely difficult to teach people how to be more creative. The reason for that is because creativity isn't a skill; it's a consequence of a state of mind. Flow is that state of mind which allows us to be creative.'

Mark continues: 'If I want to be creative, I have to consciously create time and space to get into a flow state. It doesn't happen by chance. The point is that it has huge consequences for creativity. In flow, we are far less critical of ourselves, our ability to recognise patterns shoots up **and all that helps us unlock creativity.**'

Flow and creativity

Flow is considered the deepest form of attention that human beings can offer. It is a state in which we get out of our logical brains and mind chatter, we lose track of time and are immersed in a task. We balance the two rhythms, which results in enhanced creativity and optimal performance, among other things.

THREE STEPS INTO A FLOW STATE
1. Choose one goal. Flow takes all your mental energy, deployed deliberately in one direction.
2. That goal needs to be meaningful to you – you can't flow into a goal that you don't care about.
3. It helps if what you are doing is at the edge of your abilities; take what you like doing a step further, make it a bit more challenging.

Also make sure you are following the five rituals from Chapter 4.

An amoeba is a small, jelly-like, highly adaptable cell found in oceans, streams, lakes and wet soil. Sometimes I like to think of myself as an amoeba during a creative process or when I am going through changes in my life. I find it amusing to think of myself in this way. It helps me not to take life too seriously and, strangely, makes me feel less alone in the world – I am one with the amoeba! It also turns out to be a pretty good description of what is going on with us during such transitions.

Amoebas are able to expand and leak in different directions in order to explore their environment and do what they need to do to survive. They then contract back into a denser shape, sometimes the shape of a ball. Likewise, I imagine myself repeatedly reaching out and shrinking back, testing the waters and balancing my keel until something feels right.

The word amoeba is derived from the Greek word *amoibe*, which means 'change'. A process of transition or creation often feels like one step forward and two steps back, or a day of clarity and energy blast and then a day of wondering if I've totally lost it. With experience I have learned that these nerve-wracking, in-between emotions are okay, and that they actually play an important role in creativity and any sort of transition. Trusting the process is key. We are all constantly testing out and finding our new shape. Given that the world is a dynamic place and so is life, feeling aligned takes frequent checking-in and shape-finding. Our sense of purpose or direction can change with time because we and our environment change. We need to sharpen our inner compass needle like a pencil; the sharper it is, the clearer the outcome. And, unlike a pencil, we can sharpen our inner compass endlessly because it's infinite.

The amoeba metaphor is just another way to describe the rhythmic ways we interact with the world around us. The two rhythms help us to mindfully balance the intuitive and deliberate, the creative and rational, flow and silos, big picture versus zooming into details. They also remind us to fill our tank before it gets empty, and recharge our body battery because we cannot burn our candle at both ends without running out of energy. Imbalanced rhythms can dim our light and make us feel lost.

At the heart of outstanding achievements, ideas and everyday insights is intuition. Things come together in your mind, and you join the dots. You say to yourself, 'Aha! I see what to do.' We see these intuitive leaps in every sphere of life, from the decisions we make in our personal lives to the story behind the founding of Microsoft, from Copernicus to Marina Abramović to Martin Luther King. The world is full of such stories, some untold and some told in books like *The Eureka Factor* (2015) by

John Kounios and Mark Beeman, or *Stategic Intuition* by William Duggan (2013).

Getting more mindful and discplined about harnessing these rhythms helps us become aware of what happens before the 'Aha!' moment. It improves both modes of thought, and we begin to harness them together more effectively and mindfully as we generate decisions and ideas. It's a give-and-take process. And the more we give, the more we can take in. We can't just give, it will drain us, we also need to be open to receiving. Creativity is – first and foremost – a state of mind, a way of being, that comes with the way we pay attention and what we do with the stuff our attention picks up. The strongest, most beautiful flowers grow from well-attended soil.

The inner and outer ocean

It is pure bliss. The ocean inside and outside become the same.

ENRIC SALA, MARINE BIOLOGIST AND OCEAN EXPLORER

As we read in Chapter 3, National Geographic Explorer-in-Residence Enric Sala left a university position to get closer to his real passion, the ocean. In academia, he felt disconnected from marine life, as if he was writing an obituary about the oceans of the world. Enric Sala founded and leads the Pristine Seas project at the National Geographic Society, a project that combines exploration, research and media to inspire country leaders to protect the last wild places in the ocean. Since he resigned from his university position, he has spent most of his time immersed in the ocean, to be one with it in order to understand it better. 'My time in the ocean has helped me enormously to develop my intuition about what's wrong with the ocean today and how to bring it back,' he said in the documentary film *Innsæi*.

'InnSæi comes with the experience and knowledge we internalise. As long as we are open to it, curious and excited to learn, the deeper our InnSæi becomes,' he explained when I interviewed him for this book. 'It's like when I went diving for the first time, I was so excited I sucked up my whole oxygen tank in 15 minutes. Now when I dive, I don't have to think about it, I just jump into the water with my gear and it has become a part of my body. It's the same with InnSæi,' he said, reminding us that the calmer we are, the more open our senses are. We allow the world to come to us and we are open to experiencing moments of awe.

'Today, I am one with the ocean,' he finished, 'perfectly stable floating, diving. I don't feel the difference between myself and the ocean, not even in the temperature. It is pure bliss. The ocean inside and outside become the same.' What a beautiful description of a sense of belonging.

When Enric Sala is not diving or sailing, he spends his time on dry land, planning, strategising, and lobbying with his team at the Pristine Seas project to protect complex oceanic ecosystems to ensure a more sustainable use of the ocean's natural resources. Earlier in his career, he believed it would be enough if people knew the scientific facts about the deteriorating ecosystems in the ocean, but he was wrong. What he realised was that people needed to experience, see and feel it for themselves. It was not enough to know it rationally. Enric Sala and his team of scientists, filmmakers and policy experts have travelled all over the world to inspire the creation of protected marine areas. They enable national leaders to witness with their own eyes the destruction of the ocean and what it looks like when flourishing, and support them when they decide to protect it.

In his book *The Nature of Nature: Why We Need the Wild* (2020), Enric Sala explains why the preservation and recovery of wild nature is not only economically practical but essential to our survival. The understanding that change starts from within is deeply engrained in his work and perspective:

The atoms in our bodies were created billions of years ago and assembled in ourselves. We now know that and at the same time, we are observing the universe. It really is a miracle. When you understand this, you understand that change has to start with you. All my perceptions of the world are in my mind. How I respond to the world is also in my mind. The Earth goes around the sun, we cannot change that. But we can all change the way we interact with other beings, interpret and react to the world. It is up to us to decide what to do with the time we are given.

Coming home to our bodies

In late 2019 my battery was running low after an intensive year at work and I decided to join a friend for a week-long yoga retreat at the Kripalu Yoga Center in the US. My friend had told me about her mentor, Angela Farmer, who was among the yoga instructors at the retreat and she said I must meet her. When Angela Farmer entered the room on the first morning, she filled the space with her gentle, grounded energy. She was 81 years old at the time and I remember thinking she looked like a wise, strong and slender tree. Her long legs, graceful hands and wavy grey hair, and her beautiful, big, light blue eyes, drew us in as she spoke timeless truths in the simple, eloquent language which only the wise can do. Angela's work revolves around helping people like you and me come home to ourselves through our bodies. We need to practise this all our lives because our minds often tend to wander off and disconnect from our bodies.

During the few days I spent at the retreat, I was reminded of how fundamental our body's health is to our energy and mindset. I witnessed my nerves calming down and my joints loosening up, my mind clearing and my sense of positivity and agency returning. When I first arrived there, I was anti-social, grumpy and tense and, as I write this, I feel grateful that my friend tolerated me for the first couple of days. Over the course of a week at the retreat, I watched the participants release back, hip, joint pains and headaches that they had suffered from for years.

When I interviewed Angela for this book and told her about InnSæi, she spoke about personal and collective pain and darkness which she believes many people in the world are going through now, because there is so much disruption and turbulence going on, with climate change, pandemics, conflict, technological revolutions, distractions and social unrest. She said we should pay attention to our pain instead of numbing it with distraction, medication or drugs. 'It is important not to numb the pain we may feel in our bodies, we can only grow through it if we dare to listen and own the pain.' She spoke of the body as being beautiful and authentic and said that we not only need to acknowledge it, but also be one with it. 'You cannot deny your body, the past is all knotted inside us. Meet these places in your body where you are knotted, where there is pain, befriend them, unwind them, and let them unwind. Every time we stretch and open up the spaces in our bodies, we start to uncover ourselves and come home to ourselves,' she said.

For Angela Farmer, practising yoga is 'a journey of the self, to the self, through the self.' She adds, 'Some people have the ability and strength to do big things, but I think if we do things inside ourselves, they can become pretty big.'

The transformative power of awe

The only true voyage of discovery...would be not to visit strange lands but to possess other eyes.

MARCEL PROUST, *LA PRISONNIÈRE* (THE CAPTIVE), 1923

I have left the discussion of awe until now, because it brings together so much of what this book is about. Awe is the emotion we feel when we are confronted with something so vast that it dwarfs us; it stops our thoughts, and we lose ourselves in the moment. Awe is an emotion that transcends our understanding of the world. It combines amazement with an edge of fear and we are forced to give in to mystery, to acknowledge how much there is that is beyond our understanding. It brings tears to our eyes, we feel goosebumps, we gasp or feel our bodies tingling when we witness a child walk for the first time or a powerful leader speak their truth. Our whole body is engaged in awe, which can also be aroused by an act of sacrifice or virtuosity, or an incredible natural landscape, like a forest, glacier, desert or ocean. But, according to Jo Marchant, in her book *The Human Cosmos* (2020), one of the most reliable and commonly used methods to inspire awe in research studies is to show people a starry sky. So we're back to the stars – we are made of stardust, and the cosmos is both within us and around us.

Until about 15 years ago there was no science of awe. Scientists were focused on studying emotions like fear and disgust, which seemed essential to human survival. But with the work of people like Dr Dacher Keltner at the University of California, Berkeley, author of *Awe: The New Science of Everyday Wonder and How it Can Transform Your Life* (2023), we have realised that awe is also a driver of human evolution. We've survived thanks to our capacity to cooperate like mycelium, form communities, and create cultures that strengthen our sense of shared identity. These are all actions and narratives that are sparked and spurred by awe.

Research shows that we are suffering from awe deprivation. This is serious because feeling awe makes us better people, it brings our soul's rhythms and intellectual capacities into balance, aligns us to our InnSæi and brings out the best in us as human beings. It helps us use the body and brain together in a more holistic way, and we become happier and less stressed. Awe gives us a 'big picture perspective', reminding us that we are a part of a bigger whole.

Studies have shown that awe can help us focus on the now and improve our memory. Feeling awe also translates into physical effects and activates the parasympathetic nervous system, which calms the fight-or-flight response. When we are in awe, we show more interest, we are more creative, more curious and pay better attention; we are also happier and less stressed, even weeks later. When in awe, we take more ethical decisions, care less about money and more about the planet. Awe shifts our perspective away from ourselves and onto the wider context, to the planet, to bigger things. It turns out that even mild awe, as triggered in lab experiments, can significantly change our mood and behaviour. Looking at awe-inspiring images seems to break habitual patterns of thinking, making people more creative, and more interested in the world.

When we are 'in awe', the brain reduces our sense of self, there is more flow between parts of the brain, and our creativity and flexible thinking are enhanced. According to Jo Marchant and researchers like Dr Dacher Keltner, this may be why such states can trigger long-lasting changes in attitudes and personality, something that may be unusual for adults. What's more, such states may help to reverse rigid patterns of thinking that we develop throughout our lives, which may hold back our divergent and creative thinking capacities. Scientists have suggested that awe, working through the neurotransmitter serotonin, can loosen those rigid patterns and chains in our brains. In short, feeling awe can transform how we think about other beings, ourselves and planet Earth. What a beautiful way to shift our mindsets.

Nature, the arts, culture, spiritualism and meditation are some of the things that bring out emotions of awe in us, but in many ways we seriously undervalue them. Because of the way we live, consume and define value, natural diversity, ecosystems and wildernesses are deteriorating or completely vanishing globally at rates unprecedented in human history.

In his book *Value(s)*, published in 2021, Mark Carney, former governor of the Bank of Canada and Bank of England, argues that the way our economy conceptualises value is standing in the way of a sustainable world. Carney cites Oscar Wilde, who said that we seem to know 'the price of everything but the value of nothing'; and Mark Carney writes about the narrowness of our vision and the poverty of our perspective, which detracts from our collective well-being. He takes as an example the 'two Amazons': the company on the one hand and the rainforest on the other. The Amazon corporation's 1.5 trillion USD equity valuation reflects the market's judgement that the company will be very profitable for a very long time. Meanwhile, in contrast, it is only once the rainforest is cleared and a cattle herd or soya plantation is placed on the newly opened land that the Amazon region begins to have market value. The costs to the climate and biodiversity of destroying the rainforest don't appear on any ledger but they are no less real.

Around 1 million animal and plant species are now threatened with extinction, which is more than ever before in human history, according to a 2019 UN report on biodiversity and ecosystem services. Humans and our domesticated livestock make up 96 per cent of the total biomass of all mammals on land. Only 4 per cent are wild animals. The fundamental interconnected web of life on Earth is getting smaller and increasingly frayed and, at the same time, a smaller proportion of humans have direct access to nature's wonders. There are many reasons for this, but in some places most of us cannot even see stars in the night sky anymore. 'Today, as light pollution envelops our planet, the stars are almost gone. Instead of thousands being visible on a dark night, in today's cities we see only a few dozen. Most people in the United States and Europe can no longer see the Milky Way at all. It is a catastrophic erosion of natural heritage: the obliteration of our connection with our galaxy and the wider universe,' writes Jo Marchant in *The Human Cosmos*.

Researchers have warned that we are depriving ourselves of the chance to lose ourselves in the vastness and beauty of the world, and awe deprivation is making us more selfish, materialistic and narcissistic. It also reduces our ability to see the big picture and the magic that is constantly taking place before our very eyes.

Practise serendipity

Serendipity is the opposite of narrow focus thinking, where you concentrate your mind upon an objective or goal to the exclusion of all else. It invites you to have a wide span of attention, wide enough to notice something of significance even though it is apparently irrelevant or useless to you at present. 'Serendipity means finding valuable and agreeable ideas or things – or people – when you are not consciously seeking them,' explains John Adair in his classic book *The Art of Creative Thinking* (2007).

HERE ARE A FEW WAYS TO PRACTISE SERENDIPITY:

- See strangers as messengers. Whether you speak to them or not, observe them, or say hi and smile. If someone wants to speak to you on a bus or train, or when you're queuing for the till at a supermarket, engage. Everyone's a messenger. Jot down in your journal what took place and notice how you noticed the interaction.
- Take an unexpected route, whether you are travelling physically or mentally. Taking a different route from the one you usually take will refresh your perception and your thinking.
- Widen your span of attention to include the unusual and unexpected. Being overly organised, and planning your life down to the last detail, is the antidote to creativity. Chaos often breeds ideas and new connections. Chance favours the mind that's prepared for the unexpected.

You are more likely to be serendipitous if you are curious, have a wide span of attention and a broad range of interests.

To live is the rarest thing in the world

To live is the rarest thing in the world.
Most people just exist.
OSCAR WILDE, FROM HIS ESSAY 'THE SOUL OF MAN
UNDER SOCIALISM' (1891)

'It is so beautiful!' exclaimed the Soviet cosmonaut Yuri Gagarin, a few minutes after he was blasted into orbit in April 1961, becoming the first human being in space. He wasn't talking about the stars or the cosmos, but about our own planet. He later wrote and signed a message to the rest of us: 'People of the world, let us safeguard and enhance this beauty – not destroy it!'

In her 2020 book, *The Human Cosmos*, Jo Marchant writes with passion about how 'we have consistently downgraded personal experience as important source and knowledge about the world. Personal experience has been swept from our understanding of reality, replaced by the abstract, mathematical grid of space-time.' It is as if we are no longer participants in the world, but remote viewers and receivers. With this, she writes, our view of the cosmos is being swept away.

In a world that sometimes feels at the edge of reason, and more divided than ever, we need a sense of awe to guide us into our best versions of ourselves with brave visions. If we shift our centre of gravity by balancing the two rhythms and aligning to our InnSæi, we are more likely to experience moments of awe. It will also inspire the questions we ask, the answers we listen to, and the way in which we use the results. Here's a way to convey this in a poem I wrote:

We
engage more
with the world around us
with others.
We become more present,
wander into the unknown
meet strangers with more of an open heart,
who knows, they could be our mentors.
We misunderstand, understand, make mistakes,
have a laugh,
lose track of time.
We pay attention to what we pay attention to, without
judgement,
while doing all this.
We are witnessing,
we are explorers,
artists at heart.
We experience moments of awe,
make unexpected connections,
create cosmos out of chaos,

we go deeper,
to be more humane,
to put ourselves back into the universe,
by discovering the universe
inside ourselves.

The current state of our planet, animals and people requires a new set of eyes to see what's already in front of us. Our world is a living organism that demands a new worldview – as profound a change as Nicolaus Copernicus' heliocentrism (the Earth revolving around the sun, not vice versa) and Darwin's theory of evolution and natural selection. Both these theories challenged the prevailing worldview at the time, and shook powerful institutions to the core. This generation needs its own Copernican or Darwinian moment, but including all the genders of course. We need imagination, curiosity, a sense of urgency and love for our planet to shift the centre of gravity in the way we show up and engage. How we dream about the world we live in will define our identity.

No one knows what the future holds. We can make predictions and projections and have insights, but we can never truly know. Uncertainty is a constant. I want you to go into the unknown future fired up and with an open heart. Keeping our hearts open in times of trouble can be hard, but we can do hard stuff. Jobs come and go, and you will do many different ones in the course of your life – sometimes more than one at the same time. What you need is a strong InnSæi, an open mindset and a broad-based skillset to navigate expansive horizons. Your experience will matter, your education will matter. But how well you use that and make it relevant in a myriad of situations and tasks, will depend on your relationship with yourself, other people and the natural world.

One of the most important gifts of InnSæi is the sense of purpose and security it brings. When you are connected within, you have strong roots on this planet and your wayfinding ability is aligned with your soul. This is where your strongest sense of place, direction and security will always come from. From here, you can be generous in spirit while remaining true to yourself.

Living fearlessly, aligned with our InnSæi

Fearlessness is what love seeks. Love as craving is determined by its goal, and this goal is freedom from fear. [...] Such fearlessness exists only in the complete calm that can no longer be shaken by events expected of the future. [...] Hence, the only valid tense is the present, the Now.

HANNAH ARENDT, GERMAN PHILOSOPHER, FROM *LOVE AND SAINT AUGUSTINE* (1996)

Some of us are trailblazers, or pioneer plants, creating the seeds and soil for the rest of the ecosystem to grow over the long term. Others prefer to nourish that soil – if the soil is diverse enough and rich in nutrients, good things will sprout from it – they don't have to know exactly what their role is beforehand. There is solid trust in the process. Some of us struggle to take hard decisions or let go of stuff that we've got used to, while others are like lava flows, the brave destroyers of ecosystems who give birth to new things, providing a virgin substrate for new species to colonise.

Others may be keen to come in a bit later, to maintain the growth or balance of something that has already grown into a more stable part of the ecosystem. They may fancy being part of the canopy, the uppermost branches of trees that form a continuous layer of foliage and 'oversee' the forest. Given the speed of turnover in today's world, the 'canopy people' may later want to become trailblazers. Who knows? They don't have to play any role forever.

A thick forest canopy gets most of the sun, so most plants cannot flourish, writes Enric Sala in his book *The Nature of Nature*. When there's a forest fire, it commonly burns the upper part of the ground, leaving the soil under the surface intact. 'Within that soil are seeds of plants that have been waiting for their day in the sun, literally,' writes Enric. Time for the pioneers again. We never know what or who awaits us round the corner. Changes may be scary, but for many people they are exciting because they know they bring new flowers, trees, plants, ideas, new horizons.

Life offers us a rich variety of experiences, with both tough and fun ones at either end of a continuum. Staying tuned to our InnSæi helps us navigate and grow through opportunities as well as challenges. Mark Pollock knows this only too well. 'Sometimes we choose our challenges and sometimes our challenges choose us. What we decide to do next is what counts. It's how I think about all challenges and I think it moves the point of control from the external to the internal.'

What Mark has learned from life's trials is the value of a resilient mindset. He is convinced that we must be realists as opposed to optimists:

Assume that optimists sit on the extreme left of a continuum with pessimists at the other end. In the middle is acceptance. At the optimist's end of the continuum is hope and at the pessimist's end is despair. When the optimists rely on hope alone they run the risk of leaving themselves disappointed if the best-case scenario doesn't work out, and the pessimist's approach doesn't feel like it is worth considering. The realists sit to the hopeful side of the mid-point. They have as much hope as the optimists, but they first accept the facts of their situation.

They resolve any tension between acceptance and hope by running them both in parallel. I try to practise being a realist; that's my understanding of how to be resilient.

Being aligned with your InnSæi means you sense *the sea within*, you can *see within*, and you *see from the inside out* as you navigate the ocean of life. Knowing yourself, setting your boundaries, understanding you will keep changing throughout your life and how that works, is important. InnSæi's strong inner compass will enable you to cope with life's storms, make the right choices and keep your eye on the ball while sensing the broader context. For this you will need both your left and right brain hemispheres to work in balance, as Iain McGilchrist describes them to us, and weave together your creative and analytical, intuitive and rational rhythms. Find refuge in humour and, if it helps, imagine yourself as an amoeba that repeatedly leaks out and contracts in a different shape, as it explores and finds its way.

Keep your inner compass strong and flexible enough for constant reinvention. 'Knowledge is rarely completely divorced from power, and interpretation is too often an expression of convenience,' writes Wade Davis in *The Wayfinders*, and adds: 'Not every human behaviour must be accepted simply because it exists.' There are endless interpretations out there for us to find or share. We stand in the middle of an information storm where our attention is highly sought after; it is a terribly scarce resource and at the same time our very own link to the cosmos within us. The most important thing for us is to think, digest and explore information critically. Learn to listen within; it is your safest space in the world. Wayfind in a way that deepens your rhythms and enjoy more of who you are and the imperfect and beautiful value you bring to this world. Both people and our planet Earth need our constructive, life-giving courage; 'there is no demand for cowards last time I checked,' said Gerd Gigerenzer in our conversation for this book. Spend time with yourself and be present so that you can witness the stirring of InnSæi in you and the ripple effects it will have on your surroundings. As Hannah Arendt said, 'We are free to change the world and start something new in it.'

There are those who believe the world belongs to them and there are those who believe they belong to the world. At the very end of his book *The Nature of Nature*, Enric Sala says it is time for us to move ourselves from 'a self-proclaimed center of the world and into a humble and respectful membership in the greater biosphere'.

We all have a need to belong; it enables us to live and thrive. We live and interact as part of a whole. Interaction is what shapes reality, embodying the understanding that everything is part of a grand interconnected web of life. It also encourages us to apply our spirit to matter, to create the alchemy that chimes with the beautiful world out there, to immerse ourselves in tasks so that we lose track of time and are lit up with life. Given our immense power in today's world to enhance or suppress life on Earth, I believe that connecting deeply with InnSæi will not only help us comprehend and make better decisions; it will also enable us to see deeper valleys and brighter colours and bring a sense of awe and wonder back into our lives and the lives of others.

Main keys to Innsæi

* The two rhythms and a strong inner compass are a modern-day navigation tool for personal and collective wayfinding, which brings out the best in us.

* Creativity is a mindset; we enable it in ourselves and others.

* We can enhance or supress InnSæi.

* The more experience, expertise and confidence we have, the better our InnSæi.

* A flow state is the deepest form of attention that human beings can offer.

* In a flow state, we are less critical of ourselves; our ability to recognise patterns is enhanced, and flow unlocks our creativity.

* The flow state heightens our InnSæi and makes us more connected to ourselves, other people and the world around us.

* Being in awe is an emotion that shifts patterns in our minds, allows us to see the bigger picture and makes us more creative and happier people.

* I hope this book will help you stir the *sea within*, sharpen your inner compass and experience a sense of awe and wonder more often.

Epilogue

I wrote this book for my daughters who are beginning their adult lives and for those of you who can benefit and learn from my experience and exploration, whatever age you are. It can be tough to simply connect within and stay grounded in this world. This is due to multiple distractions (both good and bad), infinite possibilities, overflow of information, polarisation, violence, grief, false news and what often feels like an extreme manipulation of our beliefs and senses.

I believe the world urgently needs us to harness the superpowers of InnSæi to strengthen our inner compass as we navigate these turbulent times. Given the state of our world as I write this, whether that refers to the climate crisis, ecosystem collapse, societal polarisation, cost of living crisis or conflicts, I sometimes fear we might be forgetting that we are all fellow humans that share one home. We are all interconnected.

In the spirit of harnessing InnSæi, notice what you feel you need most. Is it to find inner calm and quiet your mind? To stay with your emotions and find ways to release them? To tell your loved ones about your InnSæi and that you want to honour it more from now on in your life? Or do you want to delve deeper into InnSæi beyond your personal well-being? Perhaps harness it for your community, a creative project or better decision-making at work? What do you think will support your alignment to InnSæi as you finish reading this book? Note that down in your journal. You know best what you need at this very moment. Aligning to InnSæi helps you know.

A well-harnessed InnSæi builds a more open, creative and critical mindset and enables us to experience the world we live in with more compassion, awe, courage and love. InnSæi is like a muscle we need to practise. The more we practise it, the more intuitive it becomes.

If you haven't done the exercises and journaling as you read the book, I recommend you start now. Give yourself at least two months to do that. If you skip a day, don't worry, you can just continue the day after. If you have already followed the exercises and done the journaling alongside reading the book, I recommend you pick a few key points to InnSæi, two to five tips and tools, and make them a part of your days for the next six to eight weeks. After six to eight weeks, you can replace them with new tools and exercises when you feel you are ready to do that. Gradually you will integrate what works for you into your life. But there is one tool you should always maintain: pay attention to what you pay attention to and document it in your journal. Don't judge it, just document it. Writing it down is much more effective than thinking it or saying it out loud. Journaling will help you be more present, more aware and it will provide an outlet for the good ideas and thoughts consuming your mind. It will also help you to gain clarity. You will begin to notice the thoughts, ideas, biases or voices in your head that aren't useful or bringing out the best in you. The most important words we say are the words we think and say to ourselves. Be open to the universe that will unfold before you as you go back through the exercises and tools in this book. Notice your reactions to that openness and jot them in your journal.

As you do this, mindfully practise and learn to distinguish between the two rhythms to harness your InnSæi and regenerate your energy. Make sure you journal about your experience of this, notice what you discover along the way. Share with others what you discover, it is likely to be inspiring to them.

Talk about InnSæi, share your experiences and

thoughts. Tell your friends, colleagues and family about it and ask them what their experience of it is, how it shows up in their lives. What happens when they have listened to it and when they have not. Listen deeply to what they are saying because listening is a skill that helps InnSæi work in the world. And remember that people express themselves through different languages, vocabularies, physical expressions and stories that may be different from your own ways of thinking. Put yourself in their shoes to deepen your understanding of where they are coming from. Notice what that does for you.

Learn to notice what drains or energises you. How we pay attention fills our well and shapes our intelligence. When we focus on the same things we come up with similar things. When we are in more conscious control of broadening the horizon of our attention, we are better able to harness our InnSæi and intuition. We feel the difference to our well-being, energy, creative capacities and willingness to make a difference.

As you wayfind mindfully among different views, news, findings and theories, old and new wisdom that come your way, use them to sharpen your InnSæi. Think of your InnSæi as a prism through which you refract these different viewpoints. Notice the thoughts and embodied feelings it evokes in you. Journal about your reactions, what do they confirm or teach you? Don't worry if you can't rationalise your thoughts and reactions, just notice and document them. What new dots might you be connecting between bits of information that at first seemed totally unrelated?

I wish you all the best on your InnSæi journey. Have courage, keep a critical mind and an open heart. For companionship and further learning, subscribe to my newsletter and follow me on social media and my website @hrundgunnsteinsdottir.

With love and respect,

Hrund

Acknowledgements

Life is mostly sensed and only partly verbal and that is exactly how my work on InnSæi and this book started. To begin with, I could feel and sense it but found it very hard to explain in words.

In my research, I have been intent on keeping an open, creative and critical mind when exploring a variety of disciplines, world views, practices and schools of thought, from different cultures and times in history. I have read, listened, conversed and practised to better comprehend consciousness and InnSæi and, if anything, this has taught me the truth of Carl Sagan's words – that 'wisdom lies in understanding our limitations'. Accepting that we do not know everything is part of the logic of the *sea within*. Throughout history, we have interpreted and expressed it with words, poems, metaphors, myths, imagery, anecdotes and science-based research. There are many people who have helped me understand and explain InnSæi over the years.

Post-war Kosovo helped me grasp the fundamental role InnSæi plays when it comes to decision-making, strategy and people skills, although I ignored my InnSæi when it came to my personal health. Thank you to the strong women of Kosovo, to Flora Macula for our unique collaboration, friendship and your magnificent sense of humour even during the harshest of times. My friend, the writer and visual artist Þorvaldur Þorsteinsson, who passed way too early, helped me reconnect with my creative source when I had lost sight of it. He taught me some of the key lessons I share in this book and continue to practise. A big thank you to Gunnlaug J. Magnúsdóttir, who came into my life when I most needed her help. She taught me how to sleep again, catch up with myself and what it means to embody InnSæi. She was a big inspiration for my work on two rhythms and gave me invaluable encouragement to bring my voice out into the world in projects like Prisma and the documentary film *InnSæi*. I am indebted to the actress and director, Margrét Vilhjálmsdóttir, who introduced me to the work of Marilyn French and Wangari Maathai and taught me important lessons about the relationship between artistic vision, playfulness, unwavering determination and leadership skills.

Acknowledgements

In academia and education, I owe thanks to Svafa Grönfeld, the former Dean of the University of Reykjavík, for giving me the chance to design and teach my first university course in the Business Department, based on the two rhythms and a strong inner compass. I am also hugely grateful to Hjálmar Ragnarsson, the Dean of the Arts Academy, and his colleagues at the Arts Academy, University of Bifröst and the Reykjavík Academy; Jóna Finnsdóttir, Ágúst Einarsson, Jón Ólafsson and Viðar Hreinsson for trusting me to design and run the diploma programme Prisma, which we developed and piloted right after the financial recession hit Iceland in late 2008. It was an amazing opportunity to further develop the two rhythms and a sharp inner compass in a rigorous, academic and interdisciplinary learning module, with a broad-based community of some of Iceland's most prominent voices and practitioners from academia, the arts, the media, and the private and public sector.

They are too many to name here, but you know who you are: Thank you for bringing your best to Prisma and sharing it in a way that has stayed with those who listened and participated.

My deepest thanks for Prisma also go to the incredible group of students from all walks of life who taught me so much, as well as my closest collaborators, the real shamans and facilitators of Prisma, who guided the students through the unconventional methodology with love, wisdom and dedication to bring out the best in everyone: Hildigunnur Sverrisdóttir, Sólveig Ólafsdóttir, Sigurður Jónas Eysteinsson, and Hallmar Sigurðsson who left us way too early and is deeply missed.

After Prisma I wanted to explore InnSæi and the two rhythms in a new context. My UK-based friend, film producer and director Kristín Ólafsdóttir shared this passion and in 2010 I drafted and presented to her a proposal for a documentary film in English, entitled *InnSæi*. I am hugely grateful for her faith in the idea and in me as a first-time filmmaker. I am in awe of her leadership in bringing InnSæi out into the world, her courage as a filmmaker and a producer, and her talent in editing and sharpening the core of complex messages. To our wonderful, mostly female, film production and editorial team, Sandra Tabares-Duque, Faye, Heather Millard, Al Morrow, Lindy Taylor, Sotira Kyriacou and Nick Fenton. And to the visual artist and musicians who brought to life the key messages of the film, Úlfur Eldjárn, Högni Egilsson, Linda Loeskow, Tim Borgmann – thank you for the mentorship, co-creation and unforgettable moments.

My gratitude also goes to Robert Bringhurst, Canadian poet, typographer and author of *The Tree of Meaning: Language, Mind and Ecology*; Shirin Neshat, photographer

Acknowledgements

and artist; Gordon Torr, author of *Creative People*; Dadi Janki, spiritual leader and former head of Brahma Kumaris; the ecofeminist and author Starhawk; and my friends, Olivier Oullier, neuroscientist, entrepreneur and DJ, and artist Guðmundur Oddur Magnússon who were an important part of the research interviews for *InnSæi* the film. Thank you to Sigridur Thorgeirsdottir, Henry Alexander Henrysson, Fridgeir Einarsson, Gudrun Nordal, Ellert Þór Jóhannsson, and many more for the conversations that gave me courage to open up the word innsæi in the Icelandic language.

Equally, deep thanks go to our interviewees presented in the final cut of the film: performance artist Marina Abramović, spiritual leader Marti Spiegelman, Shylo Robinson, shaman and author Malidoma Patrice Somé, Harvard Business professor Bill George, Harvard behavioural economist Iris Bohnet, and my friends, pioneer Tan Le and Daniel Shapiro, founder and director of the Harvard International Negotiation Program. Special thanks also go to my friend Enric Sala, whom I also interviewed for this book, and to Iain McGilchrist who is an important part of both the film and this book. Deep gratitude also goes to Anna Garðarsdóttir, Gudrun Nordal, Gerd Gigerenzer, Mark Pollock, Rebekah Granger-Ellis and Angela Farmer for the nourishing conversations and for trusting me with your wisdom and stories for this book.

April Rinne, Jerry Mikalsky, Valerie Keller, Sasja Beslik, Felicity Von Peter, Joanna Sparber, Lisa Witter, Michele Wucker and Álvaro Fernández Ibánez, thank you for your support in bringing *InnSæi* out into the world. Gemma Mortensen and Emma Sky, thank you for the friendship, support, hikes, co-creation and openings. Thank you to Julia Novy-Hildesley for bringing my daughters and me into the heart of the Peruvian Amazon rainforest and rooting us deeper in the Earth's magnificent beauty and complex ecosystems.

Andrea and Hrönn, thank you for your love, wit and always being there for me. Thank you to Regína, Henry, Rósa, Snæbjörn, Ragna, Louise, Selma, Birna and Björk for your friendship and support. Sigurjón Eiðsson, the father of my daughters and partner for 24 years, thank you for everything. My siblings, Sif, Guðný and Skúli, my guardians through thick and thin. I will never admit to being a demanding youngest sister but will tell anyone you rock my world. To my parents, Gunnsteinn Skúlason and Sigrún Gunnarsdóttir – thank you for the arts and entrepreneurship, the love and unconditional support.

I am deeply grateful to my agent, Jane Graham-Maw, for pulling me out of the pond of writers in late 2020, for giving me the opportunity, and for her mentorship and patience in seeing this through. My deepest thanks also go to my brilliant editors at Lagom at Bonnier Books:

Acknowledgements

Editorial Director Michelle Signore, and Assistant Editor Lucy Tirahan.

One of life's most beautiful and generous gifts came from the process of writing this book. To my love, Alfreð Gíslason, thank you with all my heart for accepting the interview with me to begin with and for everything that has unfolded since, including the passion fruits, the world of the octopus and all the cups of tea to help me finish this manuscript.

This book is written for my greatest mentors and life's biggest gift, my daughters Rán and Sif. Be brave and keep your hearts open. I love you.

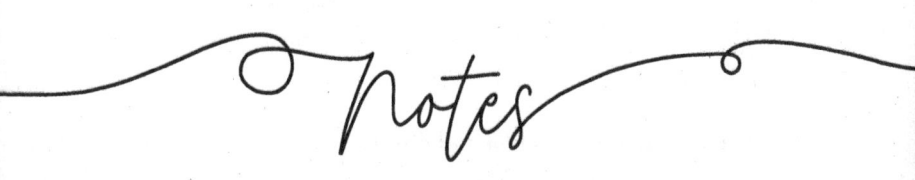

Notes

Interviews carried out for this book:

Anna Gardarsdottir, B.Sc., physiotherapist. 24 February 2023.

Angela Farmer, yoga teacher. 15 November 2019.

Alfred Gislason, Germany's national handball coach. 7 and 25 March 2022.

Gerd Gigerenzer, psychologist, author and former Director of the Max Planck Institute. 8 March 2023.

Gudrun Nordal, Director of the Institute of Arni Magnusson. 10 August 2022.

Iain McGilchrist, psychiatrist and author of *The Master and His Emissary* and *The Matter With Things*. 25 February 2023.

Mark Pollock, international motivational speaker, explorer and author. 31 March 2022 and 5 April 2023.

Dr Rebekah Granger-Ellis, expert in neuroscience of adaptive learning and neurobiology of resilience. Founder of NeuroEvolve. Chair of the Institute for Applied Transformative Neuroscience. 15 September 2022.

Daniel L. Shapiro, founder and director, Harvard International Negotiation Program. 3 May 2023.

The book also builds on findings and writing for the film *InnSæi – the Sea Within* (the *Power of Intuition* in North America), which I wrote and co-directed with Kristin Ólafsdóttir, who also produced the film, and the following interviews as shown in the documentary film:

Marina Abramović, performance artist.

Daniel Shapiro, founder and director of the Harvard International Negotiation Program.

Iain McGilchrist, author and psychiatrist.

INTRODUCTION

Cosmos (1980). Carl Sagan. [Television mini series].

https://www.imdb.com/title/tt0081846/?ref_=tt_ch (Accessed 16.9.2023)

CHAPTER 1: WHAT IS INNSÆI?

Malcolm Gladwell (2005). *Blink*. Boston: Little Brown.

Sigurdur Nordal. https://yourfriendinreykjavik.com/special-icelandic-words/ (Accessed 27.8.2023).

Notes

Annie Besant (1916). *Lífsstiginn.* translation by Sig. Kristófer Pétursson.

Global Language Monitor: https://languagemonitor.com/number-of-words-in-english/no-of-words/ (Accessed 27.8.2023).

Julia Tseng and Jordan Poppenk. (2020).'Brain meta-state transitions demarcate thoughts across task contexts explosing the mental noise of trait neuroticism'. *Nature Communications,* 13 July 2020. (https://www.nature.com/articles/s41467-020-17255-9)

John Jennings (2022).'How Many Thoughts Do We Have A Day?' https://johnmjennings.com/how-many-thoughts-do-we-have-a-day/. (Accessed 16.9.2023).

Yuval Noah Harari (2015). *Homo Deus: A Brief History of Tomorrow.* London: Harvill Secker.

Carlo Rovelli (2021). *Helgoland: Making Sense of the Quantum Revolution.* London: Penguin.

Carlo Rovelli (2022). 'From subatomic particles to human beings, interaction is what shapes reality.' *The Guardian.* https://www.theguardian.com/books/2022/sep/05/the-big-idea-why-relationships-are-the-key-to-existence (Accessed 28.8.2023).

Anne Lamott (1995). *Bird by Bird: Some Instructions on Writing and Life.* New York: Knopf Doubleday.

Dax Shepard (2023). 'Kelly Slater'. *Armchair Expert.* [Podcast]. Spotify. https://open.spotify.com/episode/7vivIqYOLwKait6wV2MSG. (00:56:00). (Accessed 31.10.2023).

Bruce Kasanoff (2017). 'Intuition is the Highest Form of Intelligence', interview with Gerd Gigerenzer in *Forbes Newsletter.* https://www.forbes.com/sites/brucekasanoff/2017/02/21/intuition-is-the-highest-form-of-intelligence/?sh=78b5f57d3860. (Accessed 28.8.2023).

Gerd Gigerenzer (2008). *Gut Feelings: The Intelligence of the Unconscious.* London: Penguin.

Iain McGilchrist (2021). *The Matter With Things: Our Brains, Our Delusions, and the Unmaking of the World.* London: Perspectiva Press. pp. 673–778.

Gerd Gigerenzer, Mirta Galesic and Rocio Garcia-Retamero (2014). 'Stereotypes About Men's and Women's Intuitions: A Study of Two Nations'. *Journal of Cross-Cultural Psychology.* *45. (I).* pp. 62–81.

George Land and Beth Jarman (1993). *Breaking Point and Beyond.* San Francisco: Harper Business.

George Land (2011). *The Failure of Success.* 06:08. TED. [YouTube video]. https://www.youtube.com/watch?v=ZfKMq-rYtnc (Accessed 29.8.2023).

Wilma Koutstaal (2013). *The Agile Mind.* Oxford: Oxford University Press.

Susan Sontag (1966). *Against Interpretation and Other Essays.* London: Penguin.

Dr Nicole LePera (2021). *How To Do The Work: Recognize Your Patterns, Heal from Your Past, and Create Your Self.* London: Orion.

Notes

Thich Nhat Hanh (2022). *What does it mean to go home to yourself?*
https://youtu.be/zqfcWWJHKFc. (Accessed 29.8.2023).

Norman Doidge (2007). *The Brain That Changes Itself.* New York: Penguin Random House.

B.G., Ogolsky, et al. (2021). 'Spatial proximity as a behavioral marker of relationship dynamics in older adult couples'. *Journal of Social and Personal Relationships.* https://www.news-medical.net/news/20211117/Heart-rates-of-older-couples-synchronize-when-they-are-close-together.aspx (Accessed 11.9.2023).

Dell'Amore, Christine (2011). 'Your heart can sync with a loved one's'. *National Geographic News.* https://www.nationalgeographic.com/science/article/110504-fire-walking-hearts-beat-science-health-heartbeats (Accessed 11.9.2023).

Heenam Yoon, Sang Ho Choi, Sang Kyong Kim, Hyun Bin Kwon, Seong Min Oh, Je-Won Choi, Yu Jin Lee, Do-Un Jeong and Kwang Suk Park (2019). 'Human heart rhythms synchronize while co-sleeping,' *Frontiers in Physiology.* https://www.frontiersin.org/articles/10.3389/fphys.2019.00190/full (Accessed 11.9.2023).

J. Andrew Armour M.D., Ph.D. (1991). 'Intrinsic Cardiac Neurons'. *Journal of Cardiovascular Electrophysiology.* https://doi.org/10.1111/j.1540-8167.1991.tb01330.x (Accessed 30.8.2023).

Thomas R. Verny (2021). *The Embodied Mind. Understanding the Mysteries of Cellular Memory, Consciousness, and Our Bodies.* London: Pegasus Books. p. 118.

HeartMath Institute (2015). *Science of the Heart. Exploring the Role of the Heart in Human Performance*. Boulder Creek, Cal: HeartMath. https://www.heartmath.org/research/science-of-the-heart/ (Accessed 30.8.2023).

Iain McGilchrist (2021). *The Matter With Things: Our Brains, Our Delusions, and the Unmaking of the World*. p. 679 about 'the gut' citing Furness, Callaghan, Rivera *et al.* (2014). 'The enteric nervous system and gastrointestinal innervation: integrated local and central control', *Advances in Experimental Medicine and Biology*. 817, 39–71. And Roth & Dicke (2005). 'Evolution of the brain and intelligence', *Trends in Cognitive Sciences*. 9(5), 250–57. London: Perspectiva.

David Robson (2022). 'Intuition: When is it right to trust your gut instincts?' *BBC Worklife*. https://www.bbc.com/worklife/article/20220401-intuition-when-is-it-right-to-trust-your-gut-instincts (Accessed 11.9.2023).

Vagus nerve exercises are easily found online. These are inspired by my class with Dr Rebekah Granger-Ellis at the IMAGINE Leadership Experience in Oxford in September 2022.

Linda Geddes (2023). 'The key to depression, obesity, alcoholism – and more? Why the vagus nerve is so exciting to scientists'. *The Guardian*. https://www.theguardian.com/society/2023/aug/23/the-key-to-depression-obesity-alcoholism-and-more-why-the-vagus-nerve-is-so-exciting-to-scientists. (Accessed 17.9.2023).

The Anxiety Recovery Centre Victoria, Australia, lists what the vagus nerve does for us and also has a list of exercises to activate it and calm our systems. https://www.arcvic.org.au/34-resources/402-vagus-nerve-exercises (Accessed 11.9.2023).

Iain McGilchrist (2021). *The Matter With Things*. London: Perspectiva Press.

CHAPTER 2: THE HEALING POWER OF INNSÆI

ZaMir: Peace Network in the War Zone. Part II. http://mediafilter.org/MFF/ZTNinWZ2.html. (Accessed 17.9.2023).

Zamir (short history and further resources) https://monoskop.org/Zamir (Accessed 17.9.2023).

Julian Ring (2023). '30 years ago, one decision altered the course of our connected world.' *Npr.* https://tinyurl.com/s7jbuvsb. (Accessed 17.9.2023).

Esteban Ortiz-Ospina (2019). 'The rise of social media'. *Our World in Data*. https://ourworldindata.org/rise-of-social-media. (Accessed 17.9.2023).

John Grant (2013). 'Glacier', from *Pale Green Ghosts*. (Bella Union).
https://www.songfacts.com/facts/john-grant/glacier.

Michael Cragg (2014). 'John Grant –Glacier: New Music'. *The Guardian*. https://www.theguardian.com/music/2014/jan/15/john-grant-glacier (Accessed 2.9.2023).

Thich Nhat Hanh (2014). *No Mud, No Lotus: The Art of Transforming Suffering*. Parallax Press.

https://thichnhathanhquotecollective.com/2018/12/25/the-tree-of-enlightenment/ (Accessed 2.9.2023)

https://thichnhathanhfoundation.org/thich-nhat-hanh (Accessed 2.9.2023).

Unbreakable: The Mark Pollock Story (2015). Directed by Ross Whittaker. [Television Documentary]. Indigenius.

Mark Pollock (2018). 'A love letter to realism in a time of grief'. TED. [YouTube video]. https://www.ted.com/talks/mark_pollock_and_simone_george_a_love_letter_to_realism_in_a_time_of_grief (Accessed 3.9.2023).

Emily Kitazawa (2022). 'Your Body Budget: Lisa Feldman's New Kind of Self-Care'. *Shortform.* https://www.shortform.com/blog/body-budget-lisa-feldman/ (Accessed 3.9.2023).

Dr Nicole LePera (2021). *How To Do The Work. Recognize Your Patterns, Heal from Your Past, and Create Your Self.* Harper Wave. Audiobook.

C. Osorio, T. Probert, E. Jones, A.H. Young and I. Robbins (2017). 'Adapting to stress: understanding the neurobiology of resilience', *Behavioral Medicine.* **43**(4), pp. 307–22. https://pubmed.ncbi.nlm.nih.gov/27100966/ (Accessed 11.9.2023).

R. Granger-Ellis and R. Speaker, Jr. (2017). 'Merging neuroscience and education: immersing affective-behavioral-cognitive instruction within the constructs of the academic curriculum'. *International Conference on Education and New Learning Technologies.* 654. http://lib.uib.kz/edulearn17/proceedings/papers/1137.pdf (Accessed 11.9.2023).

B.J. Lukey & V. Tepe (2008). *Biobehavioral resilience to stress.* London: Taylor and Francis.

Wangari Maathai (2006). *Unbowed. A memoir.* New York: Knopf.

Deborah Inanna Krenza (2011). 'The Myth of Inanna'. [YouTube video] www.gatesofinanna.com/myth-of-inanna (Accessed 10.10.2023).

Joshua J. Mark (2011). 'Inanna's Descent: A Sumerian Tale of Injustice'. *World History Encyclopaedia.* https://www. worldhistory.org/article/215/inannas-descent-a-sumerian-tale-of-injustice/ (Accessed 10.10.2023).

CHAPTER 3: THE SEA WITHIN

Nathan Chandler (2023). 'What is the Butterfly Effect and How do we Misunderstand it?' *How Stuff Works.* https:// science.howstuffworks.com/math-concepts/butterfly-effect.htm (Accessed 4.9.2023).

Marina Abramović (2010). 'The Artist is Present'. *MOMA.* https://www.moma.org/learn/moma_learning/marina-abramovic-marina-abramovic-the-artist-is-present-2010/ (Accessed 4.9.2023).

Johann Hari (2022). 'The Attention Crisis'. *Chasing Consciousness.* [Podcast] https://www.chasingconsciousness.net/episode-17-the-attention-defecit-crisis-yohann-hari. (Accessed 31.10.2023).

Marina Abramović (2011). 'Measuring the Magic of Mutual Gaze'. *Eric Forman Studio.* https://www.ericforman.com/ marina-abramovic-mutual-gaze (Accessed 4.9.2023).

Claire Sissons (2020). 'What is the Average Per centage of Water in the Human Body?' *Medical News Today.* https://www. medicalnewstoday.com/articles/what-per centage-of-the-human-body-is-water. (Accessed 17.9.2023).

Robert Krulwich (2013). 'Born Wet, Human Babies Are 75 Per cent Water. Then Comes The Drying'. *NPR*. https://www.npr.org/sections/krulwich/2013/11/25/247212488/born-wet-human-babies-are-75-per cent-water-then-comes-drying (Accessed 17.9.2023).

Ocean Physics at NASA. https://science.nasa.gov/earth-science/oceanography/living-ocean. (Accessed 17.9.2023).

NOAA (2023). 'How much oxygen comes from the ocean?'. *National Oceanic and Atmospheric Administration*. https://tinyurl.com/3m3m4sze (Accessed 17.9.2023).

National Geographic Society (2023) 'Chlorophyll'. *National Geographic*. https://education.nationalgeographic.org/resource/chlorophyll/. (Accessed 17.9.2023).

Shannon Lee (2020). *Be Water, My Friend: The True Teachings of Bruce Lee*. London: Rider.

Azadeh Ansari (2015). 'Blind and Paralyzed, an Adventurer Takes New Steps'. *CNN*. https://edition.cnn.com/2015/10/09/health/turning-points-blind-paralysis-exoskeleton/index.html (Accessed 15.9.2023).

Number of social media users worldwide from 2017 to 2027. *Statista*. https://www.statista.com/statistics/278414/number-of-worldwide-social-network-users/ (Accessed 15.9.2023).

Iain McGilchrist (2021). *The Matter With Things: Our Brains, Our Delusions, and the Unmaking of the World*. London: Perspectiva Press.

Notes

Hari, Johann (2022). *Stolen Focus: Why You Can't Pay Attention and How to Think Deeply Again.* New York: Crown Publishing Group.

Mike Oppland (2016). '8 Traits of Flow According to Mihaly Csikszentmihalyi'. Scientifically reviewed by Melissa Madeson, Ph.D. *Positive Psychology.* https://positivepsychology.com/mihaly-csikszentmihalyi-father-of-flow/ (Accessed 5.9.2023).

Mihaly Csikszentmihalyi (2008). *Flow: The Psychology of Optimal Experience.* Wicklow, Ireland: Harper Perennial.

McGilchrist, Iain (2012). *The Master and His Emissary: The Divided Brain and Making of the Western World.* New Haven, Connecticut: Yale University Press.

Johan Rockström and Owen Gaffney (2021). *Breaking Boundaries: The Science of Our Planet.* London: DK, Penguin Random House.

Johan Rockström and Mattias Klum (2012). *The Human Quest* (Swedish edition). Stockholm: Bokforlaget Max Strom.

Wade Davis (2009). *The Wayfinders: Why Ancient Wisdom Matters in the Modern World.* Toronto: House of Anansi Press.

Enric Sala. 'Pristine Seas: Journeys to the Ocean's Last Wild Places' [Website]. https://www.enricsala.com/pristine-seas (Accessed 6.9.2023).

Hokulea: Polynesian Voyaging Society. [Website]. https://hokulea.com/ (Accessed 6.9. 2023).

Mihaly Csikszentmihalyi (2008). *Flow: The Psychology of Optimal Experience.* Harper Perennial Modern Classics.

Johann Hari (2022). 'Your attention didn't collapse. It was stolen'. *The Guardian*. https://www.theguardian.com/science/2022/jan/02/attention-span-focus-screens-apps-smartphones-social-media

CHAPTER 4: TO SEE WITHIN

Cosmos (1980). Directed by Carl Sagan. [Television mini series]. https://www.imdb.com/title/tt0081846/?ref_=tt_ch (Accessed 16.9.2023).

Herbert A. Simon (1971). 'Designing organizations for an information-rich world'. In M. Greenberger (ed.) *Computers, Communications and the Public Interest*. Baltimore, MD: Johns Hopkins University Press. pp. 37–52. https://web.archive.org/web/20201006235931/https:/digitalcollections.library.cmu.edu/awweb/awarchive?type=file&item=33748 (Accessed 6.9.2023).

Yuval Noah Harari (2015). *Sapiens: A Brief History of Humankind*. New York: Harper.

'Number of social media users worldwide from 2017 to 2027'. *Statista*. https://www.statista.com/statistics/278414/number-of-worldwide-social-network-users/ (Accessed 6.9.2023).

Matthew Field (2023). 'Mark Zuckerberg cements dominance'. *The Telegraph*. https://www.telegraph.co.uk/business/2023/07/26/mark-zuckerberg-cements-dominance-as-facebook-tops-3-bn/ (Accessed 6.9. 2023).

Ani Petrosyan (2023). 'Number of internet and social media users worldwide as of October 2023'. *Statista*. https://www.statista.com/statistics/617136/digital-population-worldwide (Accessed 6.9. 2023).

Notes

Adam Hayes (2023). 'The Human Attention Span'. *Wyzowl.* https://www.wyzowl.com/human-attention-span (Accessed 7.9.2023).

Jon Simpson (2017). 'Finding Brand Success in the Digital World'. *Forbes.* https://www.forbes.com/sites/forbesagencycouncil/2017/08/25/finding-brand-success-in-the-digital-world (Accessed 7.9.2023).

Simon Kemp (2023). 'Digital 2023: A Global Review Report'. *Datareportal.* https://datareportal.com/reports/digital-2023-global-overview-report (Accessed 7.9.2023).

Stacy Jo Dixon (2023). 'Daily time spent on social networking by internet users worldwide from 2012 to 2023'. *Statista.* https://www.statista.com/statistics/433871/daily-social-media-usage-worldwide/ (Accessed 7.9.2023).

Chasing Consciousness. [Website]. https://www.chasingconsciousness.net (Accessed 7.9.2023).

Johann Hari (2022). 'The Attention Deficit Crisis'. *Chasing Consciousness.* [Podcast] https://www.chasingconsciousness.net/episode-17-the-attention-deficit-crisis-yohann-hari (Accessed 7.9.2023).

Johann Hari (2022). *Stolen Focus: Why You Can't Pay Attention and How to Think Deeply Again.* New York: Crown Publishing Group.

Brian Resnick (2019). 'Teens are increasingly depressed, anxious, and suicidal. How can we help?'. *VOX.* https://www.vox.com/science-and-health/2019/7/11/18759712/teen-suicide-depression-anxiety-how-to-help-resources. (Accessed 14.9.2023).

Noah Smith (2023). 'Honestly, it's probably the phones. The most plausible explanation for teenage unhappiness'. *Noahpinion*. https://www.noahpinion.blog/p/honestly-its-probably-the-phones?utm_medium=email (Accessed May 2023).

Rebecca Trager (2020). 'Four chemical classes cost US public 270 million IQ points over 15 years'. *Chemistry World*. https://www.chemistryworld.com/news/four-chemical-classes-cost-us-public-270-million-iq-points-over-15-years/4011087.article (Accessed 7.9.2023).

Demeneix, Barbara (2014). *Losing Our Minds. How Environmental Pollution Impairs Human Intelligence and Mental Health*. Oxford: Oxford University Press.

Hannah Ritchie (2022). 'Many countries have eliminated lead from paint. How do we achieve the same everywhere?' *Our World in Data*. https://ourworldindata.org/lead-paint (Accessed 21.9.2023).

David Rosner and Geral Markowitz (2013). 'Why It Took Decades of Blaming Parents Before We Banned Lead Paint. *The Atlantic*. https://www.theatlantic.com/health/archive/2013/04/why-it-took-decades-of-blaming-parents-before-we-banned-lead-paint/275169/ (Accessed 21.9.2023).

Volk, H., Sheridan, M.A. (2020). 'Investigating the impact of the environment on neurodevelopmental disorder'. *Journal of Neurodevelopmental Disorders*. 12, 43. https://doi.org/10.1186/s11689-020-09345-y (Accessed 21.9.2023).

D. Ruiz-Sobremazas, R. Rodulfo-Cárdenas, M. Ruiz-Coca, M. Morales-Navas, M. Teresa Colomina, C. López-Granero, F.

Notes

Sánchez-Santed F and C. Perez-Fernandez (2023). 'Uncovering the link between air pollution and neurodevelopmental alterations during pregnancy and early life exposure: A systematic review'. *Neuroscience and Biobehavioural Reviews.* https://pubmed.ncbi.nlm.nih.gov/37442496/ (Accessed 14.9.2023).

US Public Health Service (2023). 'Our Epidemic of Loneliness and Isolation'. *US Department of Health and Human Services.* https://www.hhs.gov/sites/default/files/surgeon-general-social-connection-advisory.pdf

Department for Digital, Culture, Media & Sport, Office for Civil Society, and Baroness Barran MBE (2021). 'Joint message from the UK and Japanese Loneliness Ministers' *GOV.UK.* https://www.gov.uk/government/news/joint-message-from-the-uk-and-japanese-loneliness-ministers

T. Farroni, G. Csibra, F. Simion, MH. Johnson (2002). 'Eye contact detection in humans from birth'. *Proceedings of the National Academy of Sciences of the United States of America.* https://pubmed.ncbi.nlm.nih.gov/12082186/ (Accessed May 2023)

Oprah Winfrey and Bruce D. Perry (2021). *What Happened to You?: Conversations on Trauma, Resilience, and Healing.* MacMillan Audio.

Marcy Williard, PH.D, NCSP (2022). 'Poor Eye Contact in Children'. *Cadey.* https://cadey.co/articles/eye-contact

Guifeng Xu, Lane Strathearn, Buyun Liu, Binrang Yang and Wei Bao (2018). 'Twenty-Year Trends in Diagnosed Attention-Deficit/Hyperactivity Disorder Among US Children and Adolescents, 1997–2016'. *Jama Network Open.* https://pubmed.ncbi.nlm.nih.gov/30646132/ (Accessed 7.9.2023).

Michelle Drouin (2022). 'The age of intimacy famine: when we interact with our phones rather than our loved ones'. *The Guardian.* https://www.theguardian.com/lifeandstyle/2022/jan/31/age-of-intimacy-famine-interact-with-phones-rather-than-loved-ones

World Health Organisation. 'Depression'. [Webpage]. https://www.who.int/health-topics/depression (Accessed 7.9.2023).

Melinda Smith, M.A., Jeanne Segal, Ph.D. and Lawrence Robinson (2023). 'Burnout Prevention and Treatment'. *HelpGuide.* https://www.helpguide.org/articles/stress/burnout-prevention-and-recovery.htm (Accessed 7.9.2023).

Paul Polman (2023). 'From quiet quitting to conscious quitting: How companies' values and impact on the world are transforming their employee appeal'. *Paul Polman.* https://www.paulpolman.com/wp-content/uploads/2023/02/MC_Paul-Polman_Net-Positive-Employee-Barometer_Final_web.pdf (Accessed 7.9.2023).

Iain McGilchrist (2012). *The Master and His Emissary: The Divided Brain and Making of the Western World.* New Haven, Connecticut: Yale University Press.

Matthew Crawford (2015). *The World Beyond Your Head: How to Flourish in an Age of Distraction.* New York: Viking.

Julia Cameron (2002). *The Artist's Way: A Spiritual Path to Higher Creativity.* J. P. Tarcher/Putnam.
I highly recommend you read the book and do the whole course offered in *The Artist's Way.* It's also worth visiting Julia's website. https://juliacameronlive.com (Accessed 7.9.2023).

Notes

Thorvaldur Thorsteinsson. [Webpage]. http://this.is/thorvaldur/ (Accessed 8.9.2023).

Fantastic Fungi (2019). Directed by Louie Schwartzberg. [Documentary film]. Available on Netflix: https://www.netflix.com/is/title/81183477 (Accessed 11.9.2023).

John McKenna (2017). 'These trees in the Amazon make their own rain'. *World Economic Forum.* https://www.weforum.org/agenda/2017/08/how-trees-in-the-amazon-make-their-own-rain/ (Accessed 15.9.2023).

Rainforest. *National Geographic.* [Webpage].

https://education.nationalgeographic.org/resource/rain-forest/#:~:text=Rainforests%20produce%20about%20 20%25%20of,help%20to%20stabilize%20Earth%27s%20 climate. (Accessed 15.9.2023).

Enric Sala (2020). 'How ecosystems regulate rain'. In *The Nature of Nature: Why We Need the Wild.* National Geographic Society.

Merlin Sheldrake (2020). *Entangled Life: How Fungi Make Our Worlds, Change Our Minds and Shape Our Futures.* Random House.

Suzanne Simar (2021). *Finding the Mother Tree.* Uncovering the Wisdom and Intelligence of the Forest. Penguin Books Ltd.

Wade Davis (2009). *The Wayfinders: Why Ancient Wisdom Matters in the Modern World.* Toronto: House of Anansi Press.

Thomas R. Verny (2021). *The Embodied Mind. Understanding the Mysteries of Cellular Memory, Consciousness, and Our Bodies.* London: Pegasus Books.

Hershberger, Scott (2020). 'Humans are more closely related than we commonly think.' *Scientific American*. https://www. scientificamerican.com/article/humans-are-all-more-closely-related-than-we-commonly-think/ (Accessed 8.9.2023).

Neanderthal Museum Germany. [Webpage]. https://www. neanderthal.de/en/home.html (Accessed 9.9.2023).

Shun Kurokawa (2019). 'The role of generosity on the evolution of cooperation'. *Ecological Complexity*. https://www. sciencedirect.com/science/article/abs/pii/S1476945X19300297 (Accessed 9.9.2023).

CHAPTER 5: TO SEE FROM THE INSIDE OUT

George Land & Beth Jarman (1993). *Breaking Point and Beyond*. San Francisco: HarperBusiness.

George Land (2011). *The Failure of Success*. 06:08. TED. [YouTube video]. https://www.youtube.com/watch?v=ZfKMq-rYtnc (Accessed 29.8.2023).

Iain McGilchrist (2021). *The Matter With Things: Our Brains, Our Delusions, and the Unmaking of the World*. London: Perspectiva Press.

Daniel L. Shapiro (2016). *Negotiating the Nonnegotiable: How to Resolve Your Most Emotionally Charged Conflicts*. New York: Viking.

Unbreakable: The Mark Pollock Story (2015). Directed by Ross Whittaker. [Television Documentary]. Indigenius. (Accessed 3.9.2023).

Notes

Red Bull High Performance Team (2015). 'Red Bull High Performance Team Unveils Largest Study of Creative Styles and Invites the Public to Participate'. *Cision*. https://www.prnewswire.com/news-releases/red-bull-high-performance-team-unveils-largest-study-of-creative-styles-and-invites-the-public-to-participate-300186337.html (Accessed 9.9.2023).

Steven Kotler (2022). 'How to solve your most painful problems with flow'. *Flow Research Collective*. https://www.flowresearchcollective.com/blog/how-to-solve-your-most-painful-problems-with-flow (Accessed 15.9.2023).

Roberta Kwok (2019). 'Amoebas are crafty, shape-shifting engineers'. *Science News Explores*. https://www.snexplores.org/article/amoebas-are-crafty-shape-shifting-engineers (Accessed 9.9.2023).

John Kounios & Mark Beeman (2015). *The Eureka Factor: AHA Moments, Creative Insight, and the Brain*. New York: Random House Inc.

William Duggan (2013). *Strategic Intuition: The Creative Spark in Human Achievement*. Columbia University Press.

'The Pristine Seas Project'. *National Geographic*. [Webpage] https://www.nationalgeographic.org/projects/pristine-seas (Accessed 10.9.2023).

Enric Sala (2020). *The Nature of Nature: Why We Need the Wild*. National Geographic Society.

Jo Marchant (2020). *The Human Cosmos. A Secret History of the Stars*. Edinburgh: Canongate Books.

Dacher Keltner (2023). *Awe: The New Science of Everyday Wonder and How it Can Transform Your Life*. New York: Penguin Press.

Andy Tix (2016). 'The Loss of Awe'. *Psychology Today*. https://www.psychologytoday.com/gb/blog/the-pursuit-peace/201601/the-loss-awe (Accessed 10.9.2023).

Mark Carney (2021). *Value(s): Building a Better World for All*. London: William Collins.

E.S. Brondizio, J. Settele, S. Díaz and H.T. Ngo (eds) (2019). 'Global assessment report on biodiversity and ecosystem services of the Intergovernmental Science-Policy Platform on Biodiversity and Ecosystem Services'. Zenodo. https://doi.org/10.5281/zenodo.3831673 (Accessed 10.9.2023).

John Adair (2007). *The Art of Creative Thinking: How to be Innovative and Develop Great Ideas*. London: Kogan Page Publishers.

Hannah Arendt (1998). *Love and Saint Augustine*. University of Chicago Press.